"A poignant yet heart-wa... times over very challenging terrain ... told with honesty, humour, and wisdom ... Profound selfless and uplifting this book ... [is] not only a must-... cae professionals, [but] for anyo...

Professor of Primary Care Res...

"... very personal story ... [Gunn] shares her transformation fom fear to connection and joy and gives insight into how ech of us can do so as well. Insightful and profound."

James R. Doty,
.D., Professor of Neurosurgery, Director, Center for Compassion and Altruism Research and Education, Stanford University

"I am very glad to have met such a strong and positive peson who has always been eager and willing to take watever positive advice I have been able to give. Mary's stongly positive mind has given her the ability to deal with te difficulties of ongoing sickness with calm and joy. I am qite sure that her book will give inspiration and encouraement to many." **Lama Yeshe Rinpoche**
bbot of Samye Ling Tibetan Buddhist monastery, Eskdalemuir

"Reading a person's story of living with cancer for more tan twenty years, you expect sadness and frustration – bt *Well* is testimony to the fact that another response is pssible. ... There are other ways to live when faced with adersity, of any nature, and this book is a gentle guide, wth humanity shining through."

Iona Jones,
Medical student (Glasgow)

Well

A doctor's journey
through fear to freedom

Mary Gunn

Saraband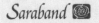

Published by Saraband
Digital World Centre
1 Lowry Plaza
The Quays
Salford, M50 3UB
United Kingdom

www.saraband.net

ISBN: 9781910192931
ISBNe: 9781910192948

Typeset by Iolaire, Newtonmore
Printed and bound in Great Britain by Clays Ltd, St Ives plc.

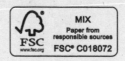

*Any details of patients referred to in this book have been
changed to ensure that patient anonymity is always protected.*

This book is dedicated to Lama Yeshe Rinpoche,
without whose help the journey would have been very different.

Royalties from sales of this book will be divided between
The Akong Memorial Foundation
and
Mary's Meals, a global charity that provides food
for children living in extreme poverty.

Contents

Out beyond ideas of wrongdoing and rightdoing, there is a field.
I'll meet you there. [1]

Jalāl ad-Dīn Muhammad Rūmī,
thirteenth-century Persian poet
(translated by Coleman Barks)

Foreword

WELL: *a lined shaft sunk in the earth from which a supply of water is obtained*
a source
good health or fortune
expressing surprise

The Chambers Dictionary,
Thirteenth Edition (2014)

My mother had a marvellous way of saying 'Well' to the unexpected in life. She said it with emphasis, mildly raised eyebrows, and a tilt of the head. Part exclamation mark, part question mark. It wasn't what she said but the way she said it. In her mouth this slight, four-letter word could carry amusement, acceptance, shock, disapproval, dismay and the most tender sadness. In all its cadences it covered most things. I said it myself, often without realising, as I grew up. Every cell in my body said it when I was diagnosed with cancer aged forty-four. That particular 'Well' had fifty wide-eyed exclamation marks and a hundred question marks after it.

Well

Odd to use a word denoting health when told of a serious diagnosis. Odder still, and immensely fortunate, to be well nearly twenty years later. And 'well' has a third meaning: a channelling deep into the earth, a hard dug hole, a space through which we draw up the water we need to live. The small word 'well' can also act as adverb; is well freighted with meaning. All manner of wells flow through this book.

How do we live well, and what do we need in order to live well? Adequate food, shelter and security are the basic requirements – but how much is 'adequate' and who decides what constitutes 'security'? It all depends on our view. When I lived in Africa I discovered that very little was enough for living well. Watching a Malawian woman cook her family's daily meal in a clay pot resting on three stones surrounding a two-stick fire humbled my own (previously extensive) list of requirements for a good life. After three years I returned to Scotland – and soon fell into wanting more. My eye was caught by the clothes in the shop windows, the larger houses in estate agents' windows, better-paid posts in the jobs column – on, on and out of sight. My view readjusted rapidly to that of an eager consumer in Western society. But at least I had learned that my view was flexible, if disappointingly chameleon. And I knew that I relished life more, felt much more carefree, when I wanted less.

When I was diagnosed with cancer my needs became focussed and simple again. I wanted to survive this illness and see my children grow up. I was lucky enough to do that. Then, thirteen years after my initial diagnosis, the cancer recurred. This time there was no talk of a cure. This lump behind my ribs could not be removed; it was too big, too central, had been silently growing for too long. Only palliative treatment was possible. I asked: 'How long?' – and was told two years at the most. Even that seemed optimistic after seeing the grapefruit-sized mass on the scan. Though outwardly calm, I was filled with fear. I felt as if I had a hand grenade inside my chest, deep in, close to my heart, lungs and gullet. How to live 'well' with *that*? If food, shelter and security are the basic requirements, I felt severely lacking in the third.

The fear that cancer sufferers and their families experience is similar to the overwhelming fear any of us experiences when, for whatever reason, our world suddenly becomes for us a deeply unsafe place; when the happy, secure future we had projected for ourselves and our children is suddenly wiped away. In today's world no one requires a diagnosis of cancer in order to experience deep anxiety and sustained fear. We only have to turn on our news channels. I write this in November 2016, in a world newly shocked by Trump coming to power in America; by the ongoing horror in Syria where years of unthinkable violence has emptied millions of people across the Mediterranean and into a reluctant and disunited Europe; by the unresolved plight of the Palestinian people; by the turmoil in Libya, Yemen and so many other countries. Our world is filled with conflict and fear.

We all yearn for ways to reduce our inner distress and alarm, whatever its cause. It is impossible to live *well* with chronic fear. It paralyses and debilitates. It is natural that we want either to get away from it or go to war with it. We see 'fight or flight' as the only options. If we cannot flee from the external situation then we flee internally: we pretend it is not there, with the readily available help of Netflix, retail therapy, sunny holidays, drugs, alcohol (I've tried them all). We put our fingers in our ears, we close our eyes and we watch a different internal movie.

Or we create a different, more bearable, external movie, one in which we are victor, not victim. We go to war with something or someone, believing the views of anyone who names and blames another group or country as the root of the problem. Even if we do not declare open war, our language reflects how often we view life as a battleground: we fight for our rights, we struggle with our weight, we battle with cancer, we declare war on poverty, we boast of building walls. Verbal violence hits new heights in tabloid headlines, Twitter feeds and political campaigns. Carelessly spoken nastiness translates into action as individual and collective fears are fanned into hatred. I write this the day that MP Jo Cox's killer has been sentenced to life imprisonment for her brutal murder. We urgently need to acknowledge how swiftly hate-laden rhetoric can fuel violent events. Our modern, interconnected world abounds with fear-filled message and aggressive response.

As the philosopher Kwame Anthony Appiah stated in his 2016 BBC Reith Lectures:

> One of the most dangerous kinds of people in the world today ... I think, are those who go around mobilising 'us-es' by stigmatising and demonising 'thems'. It's easy to do. It works. But then you're stuck with the results, and the results are that you can't turn it off ... It's a deep feature of our psychologies. It's one we can escape. We don't have to feel like this. We 'can' make distinctions in our beliefs and in our religions and in our national

*affiliations without organising them in a way that leads
to hatred.* [2]

We are not bound to responding aggressively to fear. We
have other, more creative, responses available. Nothing is set
in stone. Neuroscience confirms that our brains are flexible:
new neural pathways are constantly forming and re-forming
in response to what happens in our lives. Recent genetic
research confirms that even the immutable DNA in each
cell of our body has subtle 'volume controls' on each gene,
freshly adjusting which genes will be expressed and which
will remain dormant. Our experiences and choices in life
shape not only our neural pathways but also the expression
of our DNA. A constant dynamic conversation between
inner and outer means that flexibility is all, in both body
and brain. Modern science and ancient teachings agree that
although we may think we are fixed in our ways, we are
not – unless, that is, we choose to be.

Fight and flight, however, are not our only response
patterns. There is a third option, one that is counterintuitive: to drop the avoidance and simply turn in and face
our own inner fear. It is the last thing we want to do yet
it is the only way out. We find that when we do turn in
and intimately meet our own fear, the fear changes. The
world we are looking at also changes. It, too, becomes less
fear-filled. What we perceive becomes more tolerable to us
as we gradually open to a clearer, saner way of looking.
Our gaze widens and we are able to take in more. We calm
down and are able to discern other ways of working with
the situation, ways that give a better outcome than either
fight or flight.

Something like this happened in me after being given a diagnosis of terminal cancer. It is natural not to want to die, but it is also natural to die. I suffered when those two 'naturalnesses' were at war inside me. Somehow, miraculously, these two made peace with each other. I can now feel both of them equally, and not be distressed by the contradiction. The paradox of feeling both is … just how it is. They are no longer at odds and neither am I. It was the argument, the confusion of whether to fight or flee – when neither was possible – that had generated most of my fear. Once the war ended, the fear went. Aggressive response then became redundant and a richer, far more relaxed way of living opened up.

Unless we can meet and transform our fear we will never experience the sense of safety that is necessary in order to experiment, play and develop vital new responses to life. Chronic fear is not a given. Neither is aggression. We can drop this violence against ourselves, against each other. Different ways of doing so can be learned and have been embodied again and again by remarkable individuals. The joy of moving from fear-*full*-ness to fear-*lite*-ness came about in me because of the urgent nature of my illness. However, the Earth, too, is not well, human society is not well; given these circumstances, all of us live in urgent times. Exciting changes happen under such pressures. Evolutionary leaps take place. We have a choice: whether to settle for old patterns of reactive fear or to meet the changes with new, more open responses, and to discover to our amazement that by acting courageously (that is, by turning in to meet our fear) we in fact become courageous (effortlessly, naturally, as the fear inside us reduces). We may then find that we are more present, even joyous, and can deal lightly with ongoing change by responding flexibly.

Not only are we less fearful, the world has less reason to be fearful of us.

★ ★ ★

This book is therefore for everyone with an interest in exploring different ways of living with, and responding to, fear, no matter the cause of it. I simply use my own experience of living with a cancer as an example.

It is a book in three parts:

Part One describes my personal journey with cancer, in essence a journey through fear. Different responses were needed at different times. The initial cancer seemed curable and our children were young: my response was to go for aggressive treatment and possible cure. That was right for that time. The recurrence thirteen years later was incurable – only palliative treatment was possible; I had to find a way of living *with* my cancer and of meeting and greeting my fear of dying. I describe the loneliness and fear experienced by those who are given a terminal diagnosis. That suffering drove me to look for help of a deeper kind.

The help I found proved limitless. I discovered that although the 'first illness' (the cancer) cannot always be cured, the 'second illness' (the overwhelming fear of that cancer) *can* be cured. To this day I am amazed that although my diagnosis remains unchanged, my suffering has diminished dramatically. This is no virtue on my part; it is simply what came about over time, and I am so lucky to have had that time. I want to share what has helped me, since it may also be of help to others.

Well

We are all of us living with dying every day of our lives, yet we constantly use our energies to parry this truth. We know in our heads that we and those we love will all die, but so many of us (myself included, before diagnosis) cannot bear to allow that reality to be fully felt in our hearts. We imagine the ensuing sadness would simply overwhelm us. Yet once we stop resisting our primal, wholly understandable fear of death and just allow it to be, the war against dying drops, and to our amazement inner peace breaks out. There is nowhere else to rest.

I am not particularly brave. If the help I have received can support me to live happily and well despite an ongoing cancer, then it can help anybody. I am fortunate enough to be writing this nearly seven years after the recurrence, to have reached the magic *Sgt Pepper* age of sixty-four. I do not know why I have been so fortunate. I do not know why many other cancer sufferers are less fortunate. But I do know that however long or short a time any of us has to live, to be freed from chronic fear is one of the greatest gifts we can ever receive in life.

Part Two is general and describes the many different openings, teachings and practices that can powerfully transform our fear into ways of being that are more open, connected, tolerant, even joyous. These ways offer us flexibility in dealing with the difficult in life. We can never control what happens to us, but in each and every moment we can choose how we respond to what happens. Changing our habitual internal response from one of contracted fright to one of flexible openness changes everything. When we are steady we can look deeply and respond creatively, not react automatically out of fear. This transformation of fear can occur only on an individual basis, but when one individual's world changes, other people's worlds change too.

Mahatma Gandhi said:

> *If we could change ourselves, the tendencies of the world would also change. As a man changes his own nature, so does the attitude of the world change towards him. This is the divine mystery supreme. A wonderful thing it is and the source of our happiness. We need not wait to see what others do.* [3]

Part Three is an invitation to the reader to gently experiment with what resonates for *them* from the different methods outlined in Part Two. Part Two is like a recipe book. A recipe book is an irrelevance when left on the shelf but a source of nourishment and wonder once you start cooking with it. You choose the ingredients. What made sense for me may not echo with the next person, but my story is all I have to offer as an example of how putting new ways into practice can change a life.

★ ★ ★

This book is based around one person's journey with cancer, a more fortunate journey than many fellow cancer sufferers experience. It is a wholly subjective, autobiographical account. Yet cancer is a deeply emotive topic. Many peoples' loved ones have died from cancer. Many friends of mine have died of cancer. I am aware that personal comments about cancer, even from a cancer sufferer, can unwittingly cause hurt. For six months as a junior doctor I worked in a children's cancer ward. It was the most rewarding and also the most distressing attachment of my career. There are still children I hold in my heart but would not talk of. So to any parent, or to anyone grieving who reads this book and finds any part upsetting or inappropriate, I apologise unreservedly. It is simply one person's take on living with illness and fear, offered in the hope that, possibly in unexpected ways, it may be of help to others. To anyone who is helped by this book, all credit and thanks are due to the many amazing beings whose advice, humour, compassion and wisdom I have received with gratitude over the years and am lucky enough to be able to share.

Mary Gunn,
December 2016

Part One

My Story

One

Before the Beginning

Ask not what disease the person has,
but rather what person the disease has.

Dr William Osler

This book tells the story of a person who happened to develop an illness that happened to be cancer, and of the people who helped her along the way. It is a book that tells of loss, unexpected gains and the surprise of discovering the capacity to adjust to both. So having put disease and cancer firmly in their place, and the individual person centre stage, I must give a brief biography of myself, the person to whom the cancer happened. Where to begin? The Zen *koan* asks, 'What was your face before your parents were born?' In the Highlands, where my father came from, they ask, 'And who are your people?'

My father, Alastair Gunn, grew up speaking Gaelic in the far north of Scotland. He came from ecclesiastical stock. He was born in the manse in Durness, Sutherland in 1903. His father, Adam Gunn, came from a croft in Strathy, another

1

north-coast township. On gaining a church scholarship, my grandfather went from Strathy village school to St Andrew's University to study divinity, returning north to be minister in Durness. There he married young Mary Mackenzie. Her father was a minister in Farr, Caithness. Before Mary's birth, her parents had emigrated to Nova Scotia in the mid nineteenth century, only to return to Caithness a few years later, overcome by the hardships of pioneer life in Canada and the death of their first baby. Years on, my great-grandmother would refer to 'the lonely grave in Nova Scotia'.

Although I never met them, Adam and Mary look a fine couple in the photos. They had four children, my father their third-born. In 1907, a few days after the birth of her fourth child, my grandmother died of childbed fever. She was only thirty-two. My father was then four years old. His only memory of his mother was the way her shoulders used to shake when she laughed – the eye-view of a toddler carried in his mother's arms. My father said the manse became a sombre place after her death. He grew up in the care of his father, a sequence of housekeepers and his Aunt Donella. At seventeen he went from Durness village school to study at Aberdeen University, again thanks to a church bursary. He became a teacher, and in 1929 went out in the (very) British Colonial Service to teach in Africa.

Prior to his London interview, Dad had never been south of Aberdeen. He was offered the post of maths teacher and sailed from Tilbury to Cape Town, where he boarded a train up to the Copperbelt in central Africa. There he became a happy colonial bachelor and continued his passion for climbing mountains. During his twenty-five years in Africa he taught many children, and also climbed Mounts Kenya and Kilimanjaro, and the Ruwenzori mountain range. His great love was for the Drakensberg Mountains of South Africa. He took my mother there for their honeymoon in 1948. She described having to be given a course of injections after her new husband walked her so hard and so high that her back seized up. They were fun together and had a very happy marriage.

My mother, Minnie Jane Potts, was born in Sheffield in 1911. She was descended from families of mill-workers in the north of England. Her father, Walter Potts, was born in Glossop, Derbyshire, where his father was a weaver. My mother said her father spoke of a tough childhood, with very little schooling and certainly no church bursaries for him. He moved to Sheffield, where he worked as a baker, and there he married my grandmother, Minerva Woolley. Grandma ran their small sweet shop while Grandad rose early every morning to bake the bread, ready the horse and cart and go out to sell his fresh penny loaves on the streets of Sheffield. We are most of us only a few generations away from poverty.

Mum described how hard her parents worked and saved. Eventually they were able to sell up and move to Morecambe where they ran a small seaside hotel. Lancashire coastal towns were just then becoming the holiday Mecca of the industrial north. My grandmother Minerva was great fun, full of life, and I like to imagine a certain Fawlty-esque style to her hotel. Like my grandfather, she too came from a large family. Her first job had been to sweep up under her brother Will's cotton loom at the mill. Ventilation in mills was poor and those were the girls who got 'grey lung' (byssinosis) from all the cotton fluff they inhaled. When

Minerva told her mother she didn't much like the job, my great-grandmother replied, 'You were born into the wrong family, my girl.' Will emigrated to America as a young man, and though letters were many, his devoted sisters never saw him again. My grandmother left the mill and wisely moved south to be a lady's maid before meeting and marrying Walter. She and Walter worked well together in their shop and bakery, and were able to send my mother to a nearby private school. There my mother learned the meaning of 'But your father's in *trade* ...' from other, presumably more landed, girls.

My mother trained as a teacher at Fishponds College, Bristol. She described regularly teaching classes of sixty or more in Sheffield schools she later worked in. She was adventurous, and when an aunt left her some money in 1938 she used it to travel to Australia to teach for a year – a sabbatical ahead of the trend. She sailed back across the Atlantic in 1939 in a blacked-out ship, World War Two having just broken out. She spent the war years looking after children evacuated from London.

Her trip to Australia gave her a love of travel and she was on the first troop ship out to Africa after the war. There she worked as a teacher in central Africa, nearly marrying a tea planter in Nyasaland (now Malawi). However, she broke off that engagement and returned to the Copperbelt, where she married my Dad. My sister Donella was born in 1950 in the mining town of Broken Hill (now called Kabwe) in Zambia. My mother, now aged thirty-nine, had a lengthy first labour before delivering 'a gift from heaven of ten pounds seven', as one telegram read. Two years later I was born, as my mother liked to boast, in Clement Attlee's

London drawing room. The Prime Minister wasn't home at the time, having sold the house, which had then been turned into a private nursing home. Mum had lost the baby boy she was carrying the year before, so my parents arranged to return to London for my – as it turned out, uncomplicated – birth. My father would later tease me that my birth cost him a small fortune. This surprised me, as I had grown up hearing Mum tell friends 'Mary was born on leave' – in those days of Empire, the Colonial Office paid for teachers in Africa to return home on leave by boat every four years. Being born 'on leave' had always sounded to me somewhat careless.

Mum loved it when Dad's promotion to Inspector of Schools upgraded them to first-class cabins. However, I was born before such heady times, and at the grand age of three months set sail for Africa in economy class. Mum said the array of bare ship's pipes filling one wall of our steerage cabin was great for drying nappies on, adding, 'And we used to bath you in the ship's bread bin!' Apparently, at one point I also rolled from top bunk to cabin floor. I wonder that I survived my first sea voyage.

We lived in Africa until 1954 when my father, always wise, sensed the winds of change early. With their shared love of travel my parents chose New Zealand as the next country to live and work in. After three years there, Vancouver was next on their hit list, but after packing up the last crate of family belongings for the move, my weary Dad decided to book passages home to Britain instead. Thus are children's futures decided for them. Donella and I returned to Britain aged seven and five with a grand pair of Kiwi accents.

I grew up happily in southwest England, deciding at

around the age of twelve to be a doctor when I grew up. I made the mistake of announcing this passing idea to my mother, after which no future career change was admissible. I'm glad of it. I've loved being a doctor, although my ride through medical school was bumpy. I was thrilled to leave school and start at Edinburgh Medical School in 1970. With science A-levels I went straight into second-year medicine. Eight weeks later I came straight out again. The florid juvenile arthritis that had first troubled me aged fourteen flared up badly at university. I ended up back home by Christmas, ill and miserable with swollen joints, and missed the rest of the academic year.

Aged eighteen, I made a heartfelt plea to the universe as I hobbled aimlessly around my parents' house: *Just let me qualify. Just let me finish university and become independent*. Fortunately the symptoms eased in time for my heroine big sister to swoop me off that summer to Switzerland and Italy, a time of shared travel and fun. A summer gift of brightness after a pain-filled year. That September I returned to Edinburgh and this time stayed the course. Painful joints bothered me throughout my student years, but then gradually settled. My body seems to have a knack of allowing alarming pathology to develop and flourish, then over time fall quiet again.

John and I met in fourth-year medicine. John was a fairly bohemian medical student, known more for frequenting Highland bars than attending ward rounds. I was more studious but after graduating I developed doubts about hospital work. Back in the 1970s it seemed – and often was – such a harsh, didactic environment for both patients and staff. I took a break, first sunbathing on Greek beaches then working in a Camphill Community (a school for children in need of special care, run according to the insights of Rudolf Steiner) near Aberdeen, which I loved. While there I realised I wanted to work with children, and I returned to Edinburgh to take up hospital posts in obstetrics and paediatrics. John had in the meantime morphed inexplicably into an enthusiastic, hardworking, exam-sitting hospital doctor. We wended our ways through a variety of posts in Bristol, Dublin, London and Liverpool before deciding to go and work in Africa together.

Ours was a meandering, rather than whirlwind, romance. It took us six happily independent years before deciding to get married. When I phoned home with news of our engagement there was a stunned pause on the line before my delighted dad said, 'But Mary, this is so unsudden!' After marrying in 1980, we headed for Malawi. I was returning to the Africa I'd grown up hearing my parents speak of with such fondness.

For two years John and I worked in Ntcheu, a small town close to the Mozambique-Malawi border. As the only doctors in the 200-bed government hospital, our combined medical expertise was expected to cover all paediatric, obstetric, medical and surgical emergencies. Of course, it didn't – we were only four-years qualified. But before we arrived, there had been no doctor at all at that hospital so we simply did our best. Patients were remarkably resilient and the universe was kind to us as the hospital was staffed with excellent Malawian clinical officers and nurses (both locally trained) who gave us great support. We often operated with a helpful theatre nurse standing beside us holding up a copy of Bailey and Love, the surgical bible of the time, for us to read as we nervously opened an abdomen. We also had to accommodate the many sick people who made their way over the border from war-torn Mozambique. Then, as now, civil war pushed a country's people across neighbouring borders. I remember one dignified elderly Mozambican lady with a broken femur, carried many miles to our hospital on a makeshift stretcher. She healed well in hospital on traction, but on discharge our ambulance could take her only as far as the Mozambican border. Any further and the warring parties in Mozambique would have commandeered the vehicle. We had to watch her hobble homewards with her stick, waving her thanks to us as she went.

Supplies of petrol for our two ambulances, and paraffin for the vaccine fridges in the twenty rural health centres, were erratic since all fuel tankers to land-locked Malawi had to drive through embattled Mozambique. There was no electricity supply outside Ntcheu, so a national paraffin shortage resulted in no refrigeration for life-saving vaccines in the rural centres. Mothers would faithfully bring their children to be vaccinated at local centres, often to find no vaccines available. The walk to Ntcheu hospital, where the vaccine was available, would have taken them days. So, as a result of a war in a neighbouring country, our ward was often full of children suffering from measles, and measles is a killer in Africa. It was heartbreaking to see.

There were few cars in our rural area. Whenever a rare fuel tanker (sometimes bearing bullet marks) showed up at the only petrol station, the long queue that formed was of people, not cars. Armed with all manner of plastic containers, local people would wait patiently in line for hours simply to buy a litre of paraffin with which to light their lamps and stoves. This graceful human line would heave a collective sigh of despair when we drove to the front of the queue in our hospital ambulances to refuel. They knew how much we'd drain the scant supplies available, given that we had to fill our containers too. It was terrible to get a phone call from one of the rural health workers thirty miles away for a mother in severe obstructed labour and have no functioning ambulance to send out for her.

Yet despite the constant hardships and frequent grief, Malawian people were also full of joy and vibrancy. I admired them so much. Malawian people laugh often – frequently, and with good reason, at irate *mzungus* (white people) getting exercised about Things Not Working (as white people expect them to). I didn't realise what an uptight, entitled young person I was until I went and worked in Africa. There I learned to drop my Western expectations and simply work flexibly with whatever happened each moment, and with whatever resources came to hand. The day becomes fun when you're working in a team who respond spontaneously and generously, despite limited resources, and together do their best. Our time in Malawi was such a tumble of work, fun, chaos, tragedy and happiness that it is hard to represent life there fully.

When our three-year contract ended in 1984 we left with sadness, but elderly parents and commitments at home made us feel it was time to return to Scotland. I travelled home from Africa pregnant, just as my mother had thirty years earlier. On arriving home I wrote from Edinburgh to tell friends in Ntcheu I was expecting. One Malawian friend, Peter, was over the moon at such news, writing back with the wonderful statement, 'But Madam, we thought that you were *unproduce!*' (So very much more descriptive than 'infertile'.) He had viewed my childless state aged thirty-one with deep concern, and in true Malawian fashion had decided the problem lay with the woman, not with the man.

Our son, Adam, was born in 1985, our daughter, Rebecca, arriving three years later. Together with John, my husband, my children are the best things that have ever happened in my life. I could never have anticipated the joy (or the sleepless nights!) they have brought.

Our family had eleven happy years in rural Scotland, John working hard as village GP while I worked hard at keeping sane. Neither baby slept well. John worked days and nights, as did all rural GPs in those distant days before any separate 'out of hours' service existed. The nearest district hospital was over an hour away, paramedics had not yet been invented, and single-manned ambulances were the norm. The local GPs therefore covered all home visits and all emergency care by day, by night, and over all weekends. Every third night nocturnal phone calls would pull John out of bed to attend to anything from road accidents to obstetric emergencies. Back then, the GP's wife (female GPs in rural Scotland were then few and far between) covered the on-call phone evenings, nights and weekends when the doctor was already out seeing to patients. I can remember many a bleary night as I held and comforted my own sleepless baby while answering a busy night-time phone, wondering why the whole world seemed to have forgotten the precious art of sleeping. Knowing that John worked full days even after such busy nights meant that complaining about my lot, even to myself, simply wasn't an option. I look back and pay homage to all the village GPs of the past, and their wives, who together rendered such a comprehensive service to their communities. In the pre-dinosaur age before mobile phones, both wife and young children were housebound whenever the doctor was on call. As the years went by, I found this exhausting.

As a GP in southern Scotland I worked only part-time, so I was surprised to find this period in my life more tiring than working full-time as a bush doctor in Malawi. The rewards of such meaningful work were great, however, and I will always be glad that we had the privilege of living and working together so closely in a warm, rural community when our children were young. The decision to leave was hard, but in 1996 we moved to a larger practice nearer Edinburgh with a much lighter night-time and weekend commitment. The kids settled into their new schools and a springer spaniel rampant by the name of Tess joined our family. We all breathed a joyful sigh of relief.

And then I developed breast cancer.

Two

Diagnosis, 1997

'No way. I'm not staying in here. I only came for some painkillers. Besides, that pain's getting better already.'

I sighed and felt his abdomen again, noting his fever, seeing the needle tracks at his elbow as I pushed more deeply on his right lower belly. He winced in pain. He was adamant he didn't want hospital admission but he couldn't hide his symptoms.

I shook my head. 'Sorry. There's a real possibility you have appendicitis. I want you to stay in, at least overnight. If everything's fine in the morning you can have breakfast and go home. If it *is* appendicitis and you go home tonight, the appendix might burst. Then you'll be rushed into hospital whether you like it or not, be really seriously ill, and probably end up in here on a drip for weeks.'

He glared at me, this twenty-year-old lad who didn't want to be ill, didn't want to be here, and certainly didn't want to have to listen to me. I could see his point: I had been repeating the same unwanted advice since he'd arrived in A&E. Several other patients were waiting to be seen but I knew he'd hightail it down the corridor if I went to attend to them. The nurse was busy with a jovial but very drunk patient in another cubicle. It was an average night on call.

Suddenly he reached for the sick bowl beside him and turned grey. I checked his pulse and thought, *They'll operate on him tonight, if only he stays in.* No sign of a mate, a girlfriend or a mum. He looked too young to be doing this on his own.

Time to be firm: 'Look, you're not actually well enough to go anywhere tonight. I'm going to get the porter to wheel this trolley up to the surgical ward where another doctor will see you. Don't drink anything as I think you'll probably need an emergency operation tonight.'

I'd convinced him. Where reasoning had failed, blunt directions from both his body and me worked well together. He gave in and allowed the porter to wheel him into the arms of the surgeons. I was grateful that he hadn't been well enough to walk out. He looked such a loner, I'd have worried about him all weekend.

The remaining patients were sober and straightforward, accompanied by helpful relatives and happy to follow all advice proffered. I couldn't believe my good fortune when the waiting room gaped empty before midnight. On a Friday night, working in the local A&E as the GP on call for over a dozen neighbouring practices, you never know when the next wave of emergency patients might hit or when you might be called out on an urgent house call. I grinned at the receptionist as I headed off for a nap in the doctors' quarters. Just occasionally I wouldn't be woken until morning. One could always hope.

As I undressed my hand brushed my left breast and for a moment I thought I had touched something hard. I almost laughed at myself: *You've been examining anxious patients all night. Now you haven't got one to examine, so you're ready to worry about yourself. Get a life.* But I checked my left breast all the same. Exhaled with a smile at first as all felt normal but then, suddenly, there it was again: a small, hard mass in my left breast that hadn't been there before. That was what my hand had felt. In that instant I knew it was trouble. It was too firm and definite. As a female GP, I had examined far too many breasts not to recognise a lump that was sinister. I knew this was cancer until proven otherwise. Time froze. I lay there rigid on the bed, knowing I must now check my left armpit for lymph nodes. I was so terrified of feeling enlarged nodes there that I could barely bring myself to find out. What immense relief when, finally, I checked: no masses to be felt in either armpit or in the other breast. However, the tables were suddenly well and truly turned. The 'doctor on call' had switched roles. She felt more of a patient than any of the ones she had admitted that evening. Only trouble was, she was still the doctor on call.

The phone went. I was almost glad for the distraction. I got through the rest of the night relieved to slip back into the role of doctor, with only others' straightforward minor ailments to deal with. I longed to have problems like theirs. I finished my shift on autopilot then drove straight to an appointment with my lovely GP. (This was 1997, when GPs in Scotland still did regular Saturday morning surgeries for emergencies. It sounds extraordinary now, but it was a normal service for all patients then.) It was comforting to share this frightening discovery. My GP was very reassuring

14

but said he would arrange for an urgent surgical appointment that week. We both knew this lump felt sinister.

I drove home to my family that Saturday morning, still in shock, wondering how on earth I was going to handle this. My eleven-year-old son and eight-year-old daughter were already ensconced on the sofa watching breakfast television. As I cuddled in with them, John, just up, came in with a cup of tea. He asked me how the night had been.

'Oh, just the usual,' I answered, as exhaustion blurred thought. Doing nothing until Monday seemed a brilliant course of action for now. I didn't want to think about this lump, let alone tell my husband about it. I just knew it was serious, and I needed time to adjust inside myself. I headed for bed and slept.

That evening we had planned a family night out – an Italian meal, then on to see the film *The Empire Strikes Back*. Although part of me wanted to tell John that day, I also remembered what a friend had once said about her mum, ill with advanced cancer: 'The trouble with cancer is you never get a weekend off, when you can all be well and carefree as a family together, and then go back to work and deal with the cancer on Monday.'

Having cared for many patients with cancer, I knew just what she had meant. I decided, *Well, if this is cancer I am perfectly well right now. We can have a lovely family night out as planned. There is nothing to be done about this until Monday. There is no need to tell anyone today. Our family is going to have a fun 'weekend off', and so am I, before what's beginning to look like a pretty grim week ahead.* And we had a lovely evening. I sat through the meal gazing with adoration on husband John, son Adam and daughter Rebecca. I began to hope

15

I had been catastrophising. They probably thought I was just a bit smashed after a night on call. I even enjoyed the film, although only a few bars of the *Star Wars* theme tune can still instantly bring back that whole surreal evening, the evening when I alone knew that maybe I had cancer.

'I have to admit I am concerned'

I dropped the children off at school on Monday morning and drove on to that first hospital appointment in what was by now a tale of two realities playing loudly: the healthy, happy mum, wife, sister, daughter, friend, doctor who led her life in a whirl of busyness, a calendar full of holidays ahead; and the new me, the one with the lump, the lump in my breast that stayed as relentlessly hard and threatening each time I checked it. I had told John about it on Sunday. He was concerned, glad I had an early appointment, but he felt the lump was probably a simple breast cyst. Since he's the steady one and I'm the worrier, I had relaxed slightly, but not deeply. Something in me knew.

John had offered to come with me to the hospital appointment, but I wanted to go alone. I wanted to be free to ask the surgeon all the questions I needed to, without seeing the pain in John's eyes. I knew that in a single weekend our family calendar full of holidays ahead had become a calendar potentially filled with very different events. My world had tilted and I needed to find out how to stand at this new and unwelcome angle.

Only three days earlier I had driven through these same hospital gates as the overnight GP on call, vaguely musing, *Do hope no one's too ill tonight* and *Will I be able to cover the house calls if too many urgent ones come in at once?* Now I longed to return to a land of such mild hopes and fears. So far I had only had this one weekend of gale-force fear and anxiety. I looked to the future with horror if this was to be my weather from now on. I firmly told myself I simply did not know whether this was cancer or not. My mind opened a chink to let in other, less worrying, possibilities, but my heart stayed dimmed by a heavy certainty of trouble.

The surgeon was great. Sensible, straightforward and honest. He examined me and sent me for an ultrasound scan. This would show whether the lump was a benign, fluid-filled cyst or a solid mass likely to be cancer. I sat waiting in X-ray – my first experience of being the patient waiting for that crucial test instead of the doctor briskly ordering it for someone else. This time it was my body, my cells, my lump under scrutiny.

The test was easy; the result less so. I only realised how far my hopes of a benign cyst had risen by the thud in my heart as the radiologist gently said, 'It appears to be a small, solid mass.' My inner knowing had been right all along. I walked slowly back to the surgeon's office, wishing I could be bringing back the result that would have us both smiling, rather than this one. We both knew what it meant.

'I'll need to take a needle biopsy,' he said.

Nervously I asked, 'If it is cancer, is there any risk that a needle biopsy might cause cancer cells to spread elsewhere?'

'No, there is absolutely no evidence that a needle biopsy causes spread of a cancer.'

As I lay on the bed, permitting a sharp needle to enter both me and the lump, I quietly wondered, *There may be no evidence, but is that because no research has ever been done to find that out?* I didn't say it. I needed full diagnosis and biopsies were the only way. After all, having a mastectomy (if it turned out I needed one) wasn't something I would be prepared to do 'just in case' this was cancer; I wasn't going to lose a breast on the off-chance. I got off the couch, wondering where cells were now moving to in my body.

'I'll phone you with the histology result in a few days,' said the surgeon. 'We don't yet know, but should it prove to be a cancer lesion, I need to ask whether you would wish to have a lumpectomy or full mastectomy?' I gazed down at my two small breasts, a source of such acute disappointment in puberty, a source of such acute anxiety now.

I wryly quipped back, 'In my case, wouldn't that amount to much the same thing?'

By his heroic and successful attempt to stifle a grin, I knew how seriously he viewed this mass. Black humour often helps, but clearly belly laughs about breast size were not allowed, even when instigated by the patient.

As he jumped to open the door for me (another bad sign, duly noted), he quietly said, 'I have to admit I am concerned.'

I nodded in agreement and drove home.

It takes some getting used to, doesn't it?
The surgeon had said the histology result wouldn't be through until Wednesday afternoon at the earliest, more likely Thursday. John and I shared our worries only with close family while we waited. After all, there was no definite news to tell and I felt and appeared perfectly well. We hugged a lot and comforted each other with wise-sounding medical reassurances. 'Well, even if it is cancer, it all depends on the histology, how serious it is.'

Yet, as I allowed in the possibility that I might have cancer, a strong, counterbalancing disbelief rose in me. It all felt so bizarre. I was so well. I had no symptoms whatsoever, not even a pound of weight loss. I had been skiing two months ago. Come on – get real. The threat of this being cancer was too unbelievable for even the two of us as doctors to fully take in, let alone announce and share with others. Besides, something inside me had gone very quiet. I was so grateful to Adam and Rebecca for carrying us through those waiting days as we pottered through the routine of a seemingly untroubled family life.

I hate suspense and so I carried on as if not waiting for an axe to fall. I told myself I could start preparing for The Phone Call after lunch on Wednesday; that would be quite soon enough. So convinced was I by my own ploy that when the phone rang that Wednesday morning I picked it up feeling quite relaxed. I froze to hear the surgeon's voice on the line. A tsunami of eagerness and impatience for the Right Result, along with terror and dread of the Wrong Result, erupted inside me.

'I am afraid the histology shows cancer cells.'

Eagerness and impatience left the room. I sat down. This was it, the moment of arrest, the moment when you leave the realm of the well and join the ranks of those with a serious, life-threatening disease, with all that means for you and your family. This doing can never be undone.

Disbelief and shock mean that you look and sound like you get it, and at a certain level you understand what is being said to you. But the inner recoil at such news is so strong that most of you numbs out and only automatic pilot gets you through the rest of that first, shocking

19

conversation. The ground beneath me hadn't just tipped. It had completely disappeared. Being a polite sort of girl, I carried on as if it were there. Being a doctor helped. We slipped into a professional doctor-to-doctor dialogue.

'What exactly did the histology show?' I ventured.

'It showed breast cancer ... Er ... Grade Three.'

My mind raced. I knew that Grade One was the least serious type of cancer, but I couldn't remember how serious 'Three' was. I knew there used to be only three grades in breast cancer classification, *but please don't let me have the most serious type*. Maybe since I last looked the pathologists had cooked up a scale from one to ten, a bigger, more detailed grading where I could still hide on the lighter end of the cancer scale.

'Just remind me how many grades there are now?'

An intensely awkward pause on the line. 'Er ... um ... There are three grades.'

'Oh.'

'So, if you are agreeable, I have arranged for you to come into hospital next Monday?'

If I was agreeable? I was forty-four, a mother with young children, and had just been told that the small, hard lump in my left breast was the most aggressive sort of breast cancer possible. Its uncontrolled spread would most certainly kill me. I felt desperate to get on with the operation to remove it. I wanted to ask the surgeon what he was doing tomorrow, if not this evening, for goodness sake? Reason overruled.

'Yes – yes, of course. What time on Monday?'

'Ten to ten-thirty. Just come to Ward Nine for admission and we'll operate the next day. Just to check: you seemed definite about a mastectomy rather than a lumpectomy?'

I heard myself answering, 'Yes, yes – if it's cancer, I'm very clear I wish to have a total mastectomy.' So strange how things once on your nightmare list can suddenly become your dearest and most urgent wish.

I sat in the empty house and wept, longing for the moment when John would get home for lunch. But I also dreaded it: taking this all in myself was hard enough. Deep down I had known this lump was cancer from the moment I first found it. I was a female GP who had felt many breast lesions in others, most of them benign. I knew the difference and had been tuned to expect this news for five days. John had stayed more optimistic, maybe to encourage and steady me, but I sensed that was how he truly saw it: with the jury out, hope of good news was still a possibility. I didn't want to be the one to knock that out from under him. He had arranged to be home with me that afternoon for when the phone call came, but the phone call had already come, the bombs already dropped, and big bombs at that. The car came down the drive, and John innocently came in the door from work, to a home that would never be quite the same again.

One look at my face told him the surgeon had phoned and that the news was not good. In as level a voice as possible, I told him it was Grade Three breast cancer and that I was booked to go in for the operation first thing next week. His face sagged. We hugged and held each other. Though neither of us spoke it, I knew who was present in both our minds – a good friend of John's, a wonderful, warm mother of three in her thirties who had died a few years previously. She never made it home from the first operation, so aggressive was her breast cancer. What if mine was like that too? I wept again for her and her family, and for us. John and I had been repeating 'It all depends on the histology' like some sort of protective mantra while we waited. Suddenly that mantra was chucked, never to be repeated again. We moved on to 'But it's been caught so early and there are no signs of spread.' At such a moment you grasp for reassuring straws to hang on to, often seeing them vanish from between your clutching fingers as you speak.

John was fantastic. Shocked to the core but steady. Accepting and looking ahead.

'Well, we'll deal with this together.'

Gratitude and relief surged through me as he said it. Suddenly, even total catastrophe felt workable. We would do it together. The old carefree ground was gone, utterly gone, but we would negotiate this hostile new terrain together. We would find out how to deal with each part as we came to it. For now, the forthcoming operation, and how best to tell the children and then our families and friends, was the business in hand. The rest of the afternoon passed in a stunned haze. I loved John's honesty as he paused in the kitchen that night while making the children's supper, gazed at me and said, 'It takes some getting used to, doesn't it?'

Telling the children

John and I agreed that we would never tell the children a lie about any of this; we would not fudge the fact that I had cancer. We agreed we would never hide news from them that, in a small Scottish town, they might hear in the playground anyway. But how do you fairly and honestly describe a wide range of possibilities to children of eight and eleven? How do you tell kids that their mum may be fine, but on the other hand may not be fine at all? We decided to tell them 'Mum is fine' until, for any reason, I was not, and to make sure that we ourselves communicated news to them before anyone else did. Children have great sensors for uncertainty in the home, and they need at least to be certain that their parents are always telling them the truth. As things developed, I was pretty economical with that truth at times, but we held to our promise. We never once lied.

Being so well, I wanted to tell Adam and then Rebecca myself. Rebecca was quite sunny about the whole thing; aged eight, the word 'cancer' sparked no alarm bells in her. I told her I was quite well, would be going into hospital to have the lump removed and would be back home soon. All went smoothly. When I sat down with Adam and told him I was going into hospital next week to have a small breast lump removed, he took my breath away by instantly looking me in the eye and asking, 'It's not cancer, is it?' My gentle, carefully practiced run-up to the word 'cancer' was whipped away from under me.

'What do you know about cancer?' I asked him (almost accusingly).

'We've just had a film at school about smoking and lung cancer,' my eleven-year-old son answered, keeping his eye firmly on me.

I mentally cursed the thoroughness of primary school health education these days, and wondered just what had been in the film.

Improvising rapidly, I answered, 'Yes, love, a test has shown this is cancer, but a very different type to lung cancer. Lung cancer is deep inside the body and often isn't diagnosed until far too late, so it's much more serious. This cancer is different, very easy to find, and because I'm a doctor I found it really early and am having it dealt with very, very early. It's a tiny lump. I'll only be in hospital a week and then be home.'

So far, so honest. He looked at me dubiously. I hugged him and told him that actually I was very well, and that he needn't worry about me because I truly wasn't ill. He saw the truth in that and we all went off for a hill walk. I felt I had been as honest as I could be about all that I did not know.

For me, the worst part of this whole cancer diagnosis was the thought of my children being left without their mother. The fear of my own dying, of leaving John, my sister Donella, my mum, all who I loved, paled into insignificance compared with the unbearable thought of Adam and Rebecca being left without a mum; and of me, the one who so loved them, possibly about to be the cause of the worst possible grief in their young lives. I looked at John and loved him all the more for being so steady, such a great dad. My dear and only sister came to stay and it was so comforting to speak with her and to be reminded how much Adam and Rebecca loved her and all her family. We'd shared many holidays together as families, all of them fun.

The fate of John's friend who had died of breast cancer so soon after surgery, leaving three young children, loomed heavy in my mind. I had never heard, before or since, of someone dying so soon after a mastectomy, but what if that happened to me? Two nights before going in for the operation I sat down and wrote a letter to Adam and Rebecca for them to read in the event of my death. If not then, when? I also wrote letters to John and to my sister. I hoped they would never read them, but I wanted them in place before all the treatment started; the news on this lump had been getting worse at every turn, not better.

But then, once written, what on earth does one do with a set of goodbye letters that you want no one to find accidentally; that, in fact, you want no one to ever have to read? Where do you store them? To leave them with a friend seemed melodramatic and onerous. The answer is clear to any woman. I put them in a blank envelope at the bottom of my underwear drawer (remembering to tell a good friend where they were) then forgot all about them. In the following years I have noticed that envelope in the drawer from time to time and simply left it there, grateful for its ongoing irrelevance.

With their permission, here are excerpts from my letter to my young children. My feelings stay the same today and this was probably the time when I expressed them most truly.

Because this lump is the sort that might have spread, that might cause trouble at operation, I'm having to look at the possibility that something might take me away from you who I love so much. I couldn't talk to you about that and so am writing this letter.

I read somewhere that when we die the only question that matters is 'Have I loved well enough?', and although there are lots of times in my life when I wish I'd loved more generously, I do feel I can answer that question with such a grateful 'Yes, I have loved very well', because you two and Dad have made it so easy for me to feel filled with love.

Well

If I should die I want you to know that I will have fought with every bit of my strength to stay with you. Not fighting in a bad-tempered angry way, but rather fighting and striving against the flow of this illness like a salmon fights and strives and leaps its way upstream, whatever the force of the river. The river's flow is natural and beautiful, as death can and should be if only we can bear the partings involved, but so is the salmon's strength and beauty and journeying, working against it. Know that I'll be a leaping salmon to stay with you until my last moment. And yet it is not we who decide the moments of birth and death in our lives, they are given to us.

We are called to life through love, and I believe that when we die, we die back into the unending stream of universal love that is present in every part of the world. So although I won't be with you in the way you are used to, I'll still be with you in another way. My love for you will be all around you, joining with all the love there is in the world, blessing you in every single moment. Please don't go on being sad, or feeling hatred and despair for too long. Let all the feelings that come wash right through you like a storm, and then let all the love in the world through, because I will be in that love, and there will be so much of it surrounding you – always.

I felt much calmer after writing that letter. I wrote it out of love and grief for Adam and Rebecca in case I should die, but in the writing of it I actually did what I most needed to do. I needed to turn and look at the worst, face on; at the fact that yes, I might die young, that in this world many mothers do die when their children are young, and their children survive them. I just happen to be living in a part of the world where that eventuality has become so rare that I had come to view it as an unthinkable event for me and my family to suffer.

I felt much sadder having given into, or rather fully allowed in, the possibility, but at the same time much lighter and less distressed. My children, as they have done so often before and since, drew me into greater acceptance and truthfulness. The initial pain in facing the truth you most want to avoid is awful, but the resultant dropping of all pretence, of coming back into sync with how things actually are, no matter how bad they seem – oh, what sheer relief.

Three

Treatment

'That's all fine. If you like, you can get away home now and return fasted for eight o'clock tomorrow morning. You're first on the list.'

All the bloods had been done. The anaesthetist had seen me. I needed no second telling. Having gone in only that morning, I bounced out of hospital that afternoon with the first friend who came to visit me on the ward. It felt great to be unexpectedly back home with the family that evening rather than lying dutifully in a hospital bed, anticipating tomorrow's operation. Yet the next day, as I watched my family eat their breakfast and reflected on the reason why I was not eating with them, I wished I had simply stayed in hospital once in. I wondered how many patients, having been allowed home, were never seen again. I reluctantly decided to be good.

John dropped me off at the hospital at 8am before going on to take the children to school, the back window a sea of enthusiastically waving hands as the car drove off. I walked along the hospital corridors and up the stairs to the ward with leaden feet. I had a list of things a mile long that I would rather be doing that Tuesday. A quick change into a paper gown that didn't even pretend to meet at the back and a non-party paper hat, and my transformation into pre-op patient was complete.

I didn't have long to wait. Suddenly I was that patient in the bed who you see being wheeled along a hospital corridor to have you-know-not-what test or operation performed. My bed and I were pushed to theatre by a hospital porter deep in a bad day. As a junior hospital doctor I had always found the kindness and humour of porters a vital part of surviving busy weekends on call, so this porter was a serious disappointment to me. All eye contact declined, we made our bumpy way along the corridors in gloomy silence. Corners were grunted at in disdain for simply being there. He was grumpy all right, and he wasn't the only one. I imagined asking him, 'How would you feel right now if you were being wheeled to theatre to have one of your balls cut off?' and grinned at my ill-natured humour. You become unfairly greedy for kindness at such moments, and unduly vehement in response to indifference, but it's impossible for those pushing hospital beds to always be having a great day themselves.

Outside theatre the surgeon appeared cheerily beside my bed. It was reassuring to see that he was in fine fettle. As the anaesthetist found my vein, he brightly asked me, 'Any last requests?' Drifting into unconsciousness, I murmured with conviction, 'A cigarette.' The surgeon's somewhat startled face was the last thing I remember seeing before waking up back in the ward.

My first thought post-op truly was, 'Modern-day anaesthesia is an absolute miracle.' Second thought, third thought and every other thought for a while was, 'I've just had my left breast cut off.' A heap of bandages and a plastic tube draining blood was where my breast used to be.

It is truly shocking to lose a body part, however miraculously anaesthetic its removal. You simply do not realise how deeply you identify with each and every bit of yourself until suddenly one bit is not there. I'm sure people feel the same about a fingertip. I can't bear to think what it must be like for leg or arm amputees. Initially you don't even want to glance in the general area of the glaring absence. I told myself that the cancer was no longer there either, and that felt good.

Nowadays younger women are almost routinely offered breast reconstruction, involving a series of tissue-transferring operations. Although reconstruction surgery was not offered to me, I was glad not to go down that route in any case. I wanted this area, where the cancer had been, to be left alone to heal and recover undisturbed. I also wanted to be able to see immediately if there was any sign of local recurrence in the future.

The bandages and drain were removed later the next day, and I was left on my own to have a seated shower in a wet-room tactfully devoid of mirrors. I was so grateful to the young nurse who gently said to me, 'You don't have to look at the wound until you're ready.' I wasn't, and didn't. I concentrated on my good fortune that the cancer had been diagnosed and removed early, and simply sent loads of healing thoughts to that whole area.

Everything healed so quickly that I was discharged within

the week. Initial elation at the operation going so smoothly was marred by the histology report when it came through. I could wave goodbye to any hope of being at the lighter end of the cancer scale. Two out of the five lymph nodes in my left armpit that were removed during the operation showed cancer cells were present, so there was distal spread after all. Our second protective mantra of 'Caught early and no signs of any spread' bit the dust, and the anxiety notched up even further. Radiotherapy to the whole area would now be necessary. Worse, the cancer, though small, had been situated extremely close to the anterior chest wall. During the operation the surgeon was confident he had been able to remove the cancer lesion with a margin of healthy tissue between it and my chest wall; however, the histology showed the margin to be only a few millimetres thick. Although immensely grateful for that margin, it seemed a terribly small and fragile fence between me and the cancer. Was I really out of the frying pan? And what if the unsampled lymph nodes, the ones still in my armpit, what if they were already affected too? Time alone would tell.

We concentrated on the kids' delight at my being home so rapidly. Soon I was sharing their happiness. It was summer, the weather good, and I lay in a deckchair convalescing in the garden, developing a Tenerife-style tan as friends, family – total strangers, even – came with unending offers of help. (Hot tip to all post-operative, convalescing patients: just say 'yes' to every single offer of help.) The scale of people's kindness and thoughtfulness to us and the children was overwhelming and regularly brought tears to my eyes. One friend ran the children to school, another turned up regularly to take our dog for a walk, soup and apple crumbles would be left on our doorstep as if the fairies had called. My dear friend Janet in Liverpool, herself in a wheelchair, posted me one of her wonderful, moist carrot cakes, cream cheese icing neatly bagged alongside – one of the heaviest parcels I've ever received through the post. I cried and laughed as I iced, cut and ate the cake. During that first week home I often slipped by the fridge, Nigella-style, and ate another comforting slice.

Neighbours were practically vying with each other to get my washing off the line and iron it (my knickers had never known what it was to be ironed). When John had to attend a conference, two friends did shifts. They stayed and minded me and the kids in his absence. My sister took Adam and Rebecca up to Orkney for a carefree summer holiday with their cousins. They still talk of sunny days swimming in the Birsay rock pools. My GP partners could not have been more supportive and caring, despite the fact they now had to do my work and on-call shifts on top of their own. Random acts of kindness just kept on coming our way.

My mother's Catholic priest, Father MacLean, came to visit, a great friend of the family although Mum was the sole Catholic. His sunny, unperturbed presence was a huge comfort. I told him how this diagnosis had caught me on the spiritual hop, in an agnostic cloud of unknowing. I admitted I felt a bit remiss that I hadn't done my 'God homework' a little more thoroughly in the preceding forty-four years.

Many a minister or priest would have dived in with a sales spiel at such an opportune moment. Father MacLean simply laughed as he said, 'Mary, when I come into this house I see the love between you and John, between you and the children. Where love is present, God is present. This is nothing you need to worry about.' Oh, the comfort of a warmly inclusive priest or minister, not one ounce of judgement or demand in his eyes.

I shared with him how overwhelmed with gratitude I was by the spontaneous kindness of folk. He smiled and said, 'Remember that it works both ways. You receive the gift of their kindness, but you also give them a gift. Everyone is actually full of love just under the surface, but are often too shy to show it. When you are open enough to let people know that you are ill and in need of help, it is you who give them the gift of being able to show their love.'

It was a great thing to say to someone like me, who much prefers the role of cheery helper to that of needy recipient. I saw the truth in what he said, and beamed on all subsequent helpers. Some of the 'Oh, you shouldn't have' went out of my response. I truly let the help in, with enormous gratitude, and truly received the love that came with it. I'm sure it all helped in the healing.

Treatment decisions
'You can always have chemotherapy if it comes back.'

That statement from the cheerful oncology nurse made me sit up. Three weeks on from surgery, I had just told her that I probably wouldn't go for chemotherapy, but had definitely decided to have post-operative radiotherapy. The evidence in favour was clear: women who had radiotherapy were twenty-five per cent less likely to have a local recurrence of cancer. I was deeply alarmed by the positive lymph nodes under my arm, even more by how close to the chest wall the tumour had been, so I was glad to opt for irradiation of that whole area, once healed. However, back in 1997, proof of the benefit of post-operative chemotherapy was less clear. Dr Lillian Matheson, my wonderful Edinburgh oncologist (who has since died and is still much mourned), told me they had the impression that chemotherapy maybe gave patients longer survival times, but as yet had no definite proof to back that up. Today the evidence strongly supports the long-term beneficial effect of chemotherapy, but that evidence simply wasn't available then. While sharing her wise intuitions, Dr Matheson advised me to make the decision for or against chemotherapy myself.

I appreciated her honesty and her reluctance to order me about. Events were happening to me so rapidly that I felt in control of precious little. I felt that my body was dealing with more than enough already, so I had decided to decline the six-month course of chemotherapy offered to me, with all its associated unpleasantness, and opt only for one short month of radiotherapy. This meant I could get back to normal sooner – back to work, back to having fun with the family, back to climbing hills. I had such a strong desire to get back on an even keel as quickly as possible. Never had I felt knocked this far off-course by events.

The oncologists had nodded and respected my decision, but this blunt response from the oncology nurse really went through me. Heck, I didn't want this cancer *back*. If there was more that could be done now, then maybe now was the time to do it. I went on mulling over the decision. John and I had both separately looked up the evidence. The news was not good. For the aggressive breast cancer that I had, the statistics showed that only forty per cent of women were still alive five years after diagnosis, and many of these 'survivors' were already living with a recurrence of the cancer within that five years. I didn't even look up the ten-year survival rate; I didn't want to know more. Even with one breast down and about to go for radiotherapy, I could still hardly believe that this was me in the middle of these statistics. Surely – *surely* – those poor six-out-of-ten women dead within five years had nothing to do with *me*?

John was hugely helpful. He repeated a phrase I'd heard before: 'Remember that the patient in front of you was not in the survey.' He reminded me that each individual is totally unique, that although the health of a given population can be predicted from past evidence in terms of group percentages; the unique, unknowable way that each separate individual in that group will respond can never be predicted. I realised that I simply could not know which percentage of this group I myself would fall into; whether I would be one of the women who died early or whether I would be in the group that stayed healthy longer. When the statistics are as bad as that, not knowing suddenly becomes a truly attractive alternative, and I embraced it.

Besides, I was beginning to realise that 'not knowing' is true for every moment in life anyway. I didn't know how long I had to live; and nor did I know quite what that strange look was that I sometimes caught in other people's eyes. My own uncertainty about my diagnosis was echoed by a subtle uneasiness in others. Despite so many people now surviving cancer, it remains the one disease that brings death instantly to mind while simultaneously banishing death from the conversation. I noticed that some acquaintances were relating to me differently – warmly, kindly, but differently. Suddenly, although you feel you are the same person you have always been, others look at you as if you are now in a special club; a club you did not know you were in, and one you definitely don't know the rules of. It is a dislocating and isolating type of feeling. It came to me when people talked overly brightly to me with a distracted, anxious look in their eye. I am not being critical. Their look came from concern. I am sure it is the way I unconsciously behaved in the past too. Finally I understood, and burst out laughing when I did. I remember going home and saying to my husband, 'I've got it. I've just understood what that weird look in some peoples' eyes means. They think *I'm* going to die but *they're* not! Yet we are all going to die. I don't fundamentally feel any different from them. Why are they projecting the whole death thing on to me?'

It was an impossible look to do business with. How could one say to such well-meaning, truly concerned folk, 'Don't be so concerned about me. I thank you for your worry for me, and you are right – I do stand more of a chance of dying sooner than you. But the truth is, we are all of us going to die. I really don't feel that different from you. I'm simply more in touch with the fact that I, and everyone else, will at some point die.' It would have been too brutal to be that honest back, and maybe I was misreading the look anyway. But it was a bizarrely isolating look to receive, and one that I'm sure is linked to our current death-defying/death-denying culture.

Our whole society tends to deny death and push its inevitability far away into some dim and distant future. This is understandable. One hundred years ago, average life expectancy in Britain was around fifty years. Now it is around eighty years. Our society today enjoys much more *life* expectancy than *death* expectancy. However, this means that a young person being diagnosed with cancer is threatening, shocking to us. It is inevitable that some will talk to a cancer patient with a look of veiled horror. That suddenly kindled fear I saw in peoples' eyes was simply fear of their own unacknowledged mortality. When gently acknowledged and owned, that fear eases and settles as we help each other recognise, accept and calm down about death. However, when left unowned and unclaimed, that fear ricochets around society and an unfair portion can get pushed on to cancer patients. This doesn't help. They're learning to deal with their own fear. They really don't need everyone else's too.

I came to understand that in cancer (or any other serious illness) there are two illnesses. The 'first illness' is the cancer itself and the physical symptoms that it brings. The 'second illness' is the commanding fear that nearly all cancer patients – and their friends and family – suffer regarding the unknown but threat-filled future: the fear from wondering whether the aggressive treatment regimes will kill them rather than cure them; how long before a recurrence; whether any real cure is on the horizon; whether their pain will be adequately controlled; how their family will manage without them … The list is endless. The overwhelming anxiety of this second illness can be more debilitating than the physical symptoms of the first.

Somehow, acknowledgement of our common mortality has almost slipped into public unconsciousness. How is it that an event that most assuredly will happen to every single person on the planet has come to be viewed as extraordinary? Why was I feeling somehow outside the invisible city wall of normality now that I carried a cancer diagnosis? Yet I was also receiving so many random practical acts of such kindness, often from near strangers, that I felt more wrapped in human warmth than ever before. What a mixture we human beings are. And still, this particular human being could not come to a final decision about whether to have chemotherapy or not.

A good bottle of wine

Firm decisions come at the most unexpected times. Mine came as I swept out of the ladies' in a sunny canal-side restaurant in Leith. John and I had retreated there after another long and daunting appointment with the oncologists. Tired of talking about the cancer, we were simply having a lovely meal, sharing a bottle of wine and laughing and chatting about everything under the sun. Surprisingly, these lightsome moments are possible even in the middle of grim times − if you notice and allow them. I felt light, joyful, almost carefree again − and yes, fairly drunk. John was driving and had only had one glass, yet the bottle was mysteriously empty.

Swinging back into the restaurant, the thought came to my mind unasked: *I love my life, I want as much more of it as is possible. If chemo adds to how long I can live and love life, then I'll go for it now.* And that decision held firm long after the uplifting effect of a bottle of Gewürztraminer had worn off.

Chemotherapy

One month after the mastectomy I felt completely well. It had been wonderful to experience my body growing stronger each day. My mastectomy wound had healed and

Treatment

I was now able now look at the scar. I didn't like its ragged, pulled look, the plain flatness it covered. I shrank at seeing the outline of my ribs so clearly beneath it. Yet I was enormously grateful to have had the aggressive cancer removed. That breast had suddenly been such trouble that I was glad to have it gone.

What was difficult to take in was that, despite my body having done such a great job at healing, despite feeling I was finally coming up for air after the operation, I was about to put my poor body through intense chemotherapy and radiotherapy. Yet that is the whole drive of the modern cancer treatment which has so improved survival statistics – to keep attacking any remaining cancer cells with the fiercest treatment possible in order to eradicate them. I was glad I had made the decision for both chemotherapy and radiotherapy myself, as otherwise I might not have been able to hold myself to script.

On a sunny July morning, John drove me to the nearby district hospital to have my first dose of chemotherapy. The excellent oncology nurse carefully inserted the intravenous needle and then injected what seemed like industrial doses of chemicals (in my case, cyclophosphamide, methotrexate and 5-fluorouracil) through massive syringes. She explained all of the side effects of each of these three toxic agents and I was sent home with full hand-outs describing all possible problems that patients on this regime might experience. I'd had enough unfavourable details right then, though, and couldn't take in any more. I knew the stuff was toxic – after all, that was the whole point. So I glanced only briefly at the literature. When I mentioned this to John much later he said, 'You too? I never read them either.'

Everything they say about chemotherapy is true. You do feel truly lousy and your body feels as exhausted as if it has run a marathon. The grey nausea after each treatment would wear off by the third day. I would then lie about for a few days, incapable of much more than making a cup of tea as I crawled slowly back to a semblance of normality. Just as I came to and felt I might be able to do something normal, it was time for the next dose. Initially I went back part-time to the health centre where I worked, going in only during the more normal two weeks preceding each monthly chemo. As the exhaustion built with each treatment, and as my white cell count proved slow to come back up, I realised I was trying to appear okay when actually I was far from it. After three months, I gave up any pretence of normal functioning and accepted being signed off work until all treatment was completed.

I had been warned to expect possible total hair loss and had a somewhat bushy NHS wig at the ready. The kids had tried it on with great hilarity when I had come home with it in my bag. We all giggled at John in it – with his moustache he made a scary, hairy George Harrison looka-like. However, to my great good fortune my hair decided to hang on in there throughout all treatment and the wig never saw action. I was so grateful that I went on looking normal for the children. That felt a great boon. Besides, it felt like a tight woolly hat.

It was frustrating not to have the energy to join in normal family activity, but once we all accepted that was just the way it was, the kids seemed fine with it. One Saturday morning as they left for a walk, I heard Rebecca asking John whether I was coming too.

'No,' answered John. 'Mum's having a rest. For now she's lost a bit of her get-up-and-go.'

As they all went out the door I heard Adam matter-of-factly remark, 'Yeah, all Mum's get-up-and-go has kind of lied down and flopped.'

That to me is the best description ever of the effect of chemotherapy. Your get-up-and-go simply lies down and flops.

Radiotherapy

After three months of chemotherapy (three more would follow later), I was sent for a month of radiotherapy at the Western General Hospital in Edinburgh, an hour-and-a-half's drive away. This consisted of one short treatment a day, five days a week, for four weeks – twenty treatments in all. I could have been driven there and back each day, but that felt like a Herculean undertaking from where I was now flopped. Luckily the Western General Hospital had a house nearby where radiotherapy patients could stay and I booked in there for the month, driving myself home each weekend. Raeburn House was a godsend: a quiet, slightly rundown house within walking distance of the hospital, where we-who-were-about-to-receive radiotherapy could salute each other.

I knew I needed some time away from the family to come to terms with all this, without any energy going into pretence. No matter how much you vow to be truthful, a mother tends to put on a bright smile, shove the sick bowl under the bed and engage in semi-animated discussion as soon as her young child comes bouncing into the room. I was running out of energy even to do that, and was relieved for a while to go and flop among strangers whose faces would not be shot through with anxiety whenever I looked grey.

I became very fond of my fellow residents in Raeburn House over that month. We were such a haphazard bunch: young and old, male and female, the seemingly healthy and the obviously unwell, the serene and the morose, those who went out for walks and those who sat firmly in the lounge with their knitting, those who wished to talk and those who zipped the lip. Every type of cancer diagnosis under the sun was housed under that roof. At night I could almost feel the building shaking with the hidden agitations of its residents. The floorboards were so creaky that you could hear every nocturnal trip to the toilet, and there were many. Nights were light on sleep for all concerned. Two senior nurses took shifts in reception. I had asked them not to inform the other residents that I was a doctor and I made sure that I never did so myself. Somehow, whatever the company, if others find out that you are a GP they start urgently communicating their symptoms and problems to you. This building was full of life-threatening problems and I had come with my own ample bundle. I knew I had no energy left other than to quietly send goodwill to everyone as a fellow patient.

The staff in the radiotherapy department could not have been kinder, more professional, or more pressurised. You made sure you always went early for your treatment time, knowing you needed to give the staff all possible flexibility. You might well be asked to come back later, depending on the day. If one of the machines broke down, somehow they juggled a way of giving everyone their proper treatment, but my sense was there was precious little slack in the system. As the person before you went in for their treatment you were asked to sit in a chair right beside the passage leading to the radiotherapy machine. As one patient walked out, the next patient would, quite literally, walk in. As we passed each other, we would exchange wry smiles as we handed over our invisible treatment baton in this strange relay race.

Strange indeed – to each day walk down the twice right-angled passage leading to the radiotherapy machine, the bends in the corridor there to prevent the powerful radiation aimed at you from leaking out and harming others. Strange to lie on a table and allow yourself to be positioned with great care by pleasant technicians who then focus and calibrate the large overhead machine that delivers the radiation. Strange to then be left lying alone in the large room, hearing their brisk footsteps fading away down the corridor. Strange not to leap off the bed and follow them out, away from all this carefully controlled fierceness. Strange to lie utterly still while the massive machine moves in a slow arc around you, all the while clicking and delivering its fierce rays. Strange to find that you cannot yet look at the machine, as the daily dose passes painlessly through you.

Finding other support
Some welcome respite was provided by the first of many Maggie's Centres which had been built recently in the grounds of the Western General. It was wonderful to sit and have a cup of tea in the centre's homely, light-filled interior and talk to the staff there. One afternoon I joined other female Raeburn House residents there for a free make-up session. I ungraciously don't remember which

cosmetic firm had generously donated their staff, cosmetics and full goodie bags for the likes of us. I should remember, as I used their eye shadow and mascara for years after. I do remember our group returning to Raeburn House later that afternoon, a bizarrely glamorous set of artificial faces, laughing together at our situation. As one woman said, 'All dressed up with nowhere to go.'

Between treatments I often went for slow walks in the Royal Botanic Garden, feeling as autumnal as the leaves around me. I also reached out for other help. I wandered around the bookshops and was brought to a halt by the title of one book standing central in a Stockbridge shop window: *When Things Fall Apart: Heart Advice for Difficult Times*.[1] I bought it for the title alone. I had never heard of the author, Pema Chödrön, an American Buddhist nun, but this wonderful book became a lifeline for me. So did attending gentle evening walking meditations at the nearby Buddhist Kagyu Samye Dzong meditation centre in Edinburgh. I didn't need to be a Buddhist. I didn't need to confide in the leader or my fellow meditators about my situation. I was weary of recounting the story. I simply loved their calm and the fact that they gently walked in silence, at a pace I could go at without having to rest and sit down. They have no idea how much they helped me.

Faced with the threat of early death, I felt quite adrift in the world. I believed in no god to whom I could pray, or against whom I could rage. I attended no church, nor did I feel any pull to find one. As children of an Anglican, English, Tory-voting mother (who later became a Catholic) and a Presbyterian, Scottish, Liberal-voting father, my sister and I had a broad upbringing. Mum and Dad were relaxed and tolerant of each other's different views. At election times, interestingly defaced photos of each other's political candidates would appear in unexpected places around the house. They enjoyed each other's differences and never sought to amend them. On polling day Mum and Dad would faithfully vote, never minding that they usually cancelled out each other's vote. Once, when Mum complained that she had caught a flea after attending church one Sunday, I heard her laughing in the bedroom as Dad good-naturedly said, 'I'm not a bit surprised, the sort of people you worship with.' Another time, when she asked whether he, the son of a Presbyterian minister, would mind her becoming a Catholic, Dad smiled and said, 'Jane, you could kiss the Pope's big toe for all that I would mind.'

Their open-mindedness showed in our schooling. First we went to a Catholic primary, then on to a Methodist secondary school. I was very fortunate – the nuns who taught me as a young child were wonderful, and the Methodist school Mum and Dad chose had good teachers too (although its crazy motto, 'Beyond the best there is a better', defied both grammar and common sense). My sister and I became adept at ducking out of the way of oncoming priests or ministers bearing communion books. I would meekly ride in my bold sister's slipstream as she firmly told them that one or other of our parents would not want us to join their church. She was consistent – all clerics got the same answer. I left school tolerant of diversity, with no commitment to any one religion. Mum and Dad were happy for us to make up our own minds, and we were both happy not to. If anything, I was a vague, open-minded agnostic.

Though not attracted to any form of organised religion, I did start to wonder once I'd met certain individuals, often from differing faiths. Mum's priest, Father MacLean, was one. Humility and joy radiated from him and, not being a Catholic myself, I felt free to ask him all sorts of questions, to which he always gave stimulating answers. Then there was the Reverend John Smith of North Uist, whose church I never attended, but who I used to meet with John's family when we were there on holiday. He had the same quiet, warm presence. I knew that if I had suffered a loss I would be very pleased indeed to be visited by either of these two remarkable men.

Some of the missionary nuns we had worked with in Africa were pretty special too. I remember one Catholic nun who ran a rural health station in our district. She used to frequently refer multigravida mothers (women who had had many pregnancies) who wished to have their tubes tied and be sterilised. In rural Africa, once a woman has had four or more pregnancies the chances of her dying of a complication in a further pregnancy is high – and many Malawian women have eight or ten pregnancies. There was little to no alternative contraception available and I was delighted that my friend the nun was referring them. However, one day I teasingly asked her, 'Now then, Sister, what would your headman (then Pope John Paul II) say about all these referrals for sterilisation?' She laughed and said tenderly, affectionately, 'Oh, one man. He cannot know everything.' I liked her answer.

Although I did not seek out any church or institution when having treatment for cancer, I did seek out individual help. I knew I needed it. A friend introduced me to Sister

Helen, a marvellous Catholic nun who gave her warmth and wisdom to all who came to her. When I was having radiotherapy I went to see her at a retreat house in Morningside once a week. Just like Father MacLean, she listened and loved, and helped me to accept this new, fragile being I had become. So much comes up at these vulnerable times. When I shared with her the inner sense of unworthiness which I had vaguely sensed and parried ever since childhood, the open joy and certainty with which she said, 'But Mary, you are loved beyond your wildest imaginings,' brought tears to my eyes.

As a doctor who had recently started practicing homeopathy, I now sought homeopathic treatment myself. I have never understood the outrage in some conventional medical circles against so-called 'alternative' methods of healing. I have always wanted to answer gently, 'Come on guys, when we in conventional medicine have all the answers, then we can take that line. We're actually so far from being able to help all patients with all illnesses ourselves, shouldn't we just keep a more open tolerant mind about other possibilities, as long as they do no harm?' I have also never understood the either/or thinking of many doctors, who tell their patients they should go down only one treatment route or the other. I am a happy celebrator of chemotherapy, radiotherapy, homeopathy, acupuncture and other therapies.

As I gave my history to the homeopathic doctor I sought out, it was hugely helpful to begin to see the whole of me, not just this illness. It was as if the being in whom this cancer was housed was allowed to show herself for the first time. The focus widened and I began to see all the forces acting on me in the run-up to the diagnosis, and how I had been responding to them. When something as 'wrong' as developing cancer relatively young happens to you, *in* you, you cannot help but wonder whether you or the world has done something to cause this (whether you own up to this feeling or not). Our move across Scotland the previous year, the deeper reasons for that move, my mother's now-established dementia – all had entailed a great deal of personal sadness and family stress. Had this contributed to me getting cancer now? No one can answer that question. Statistics show a much higher incidence of cancer in the year following a major bereavement, so clearly grief and stress play a part in the development and timing of the disease, but both grief and stress are also a normal part of living. Had the world thrown too much at me all at once? Had my inability to process that too-muchness contributed to my present diagnosis?

My underlying, unexamined assumption at that time was that something wrong had happened and that maybe somewhere, somehow, someone must have blundered in order for this to happen. If so, who? Was it me, someone else, the universe or God? I couldn't see any other players. In her pioneering 1969 book *On Death and Dying*,[2] psychiatrist Elisabeth Kübler-Ross described five stages in processing grief and loss: denial, anger, bargaining, depression and acceptance. She described these 'stages' as tentative and emphasised that they often overlapped. In my own experience, both as doctor and patient, these stages do not necessarily occur in linear order; the journey through grief and loss being different for each unique individual. Fully allowing the feeling, and allowing each feeling to change and move on, is healthy. The only problem is when we get stuck and fixed in any one of these stages. Even once in acceptance, we can still take the occasional whirlwind tour through the other four stages again. My wondering whether anyone or anything had contributed to my cancer was simply my personal form of the bargaining stage. My storyline ran, 'If I'd done this, or if he or she had not done that, then maybe this would not have happened.'

People tend to fall into two groups when the difficult happens: those who 'blame out' and those who 'blame in'. If you're very unlucky you do both. I tend just to blame in. As Sister Helen told me with a chuckle, we can all – maybe particularly in Scotland – be hard on ourselves and suffer from a 'hardening of the oughteries'. As I spoke with the homeopathic doctor, I began to hear how strong my underlying sense was that somehow I *should have* dealt better with events. It was only part of Kübler-Ross's bargaining stage, but if I'd left it unacknowledged and unrecognised I could have stayed stuck in it. A destructive, unconscious blaming-in had been going on. As the mindfulness teacher Rob Nairn more bluntly points out, 'You're not by any chance *shoulding* on yourself, are you?'

I am so grateful to that homeopathic doctor, who listened, let me hear myself and helped me to see, and largely let go of, my subliminal worry that I'd done something wrong. It's bad enough having cancer without also thinking that you're to blame. At the same time the doctor helped me recognise routine ways in which I responded to life, often needlessly over-using my energy in times of stress. I could certainly do with kicking that habit at this point. I wanted to conserve all energy to maximise healing.

I realised how much I perennially saw myself as the one

who must rush to put things right for others, the one who was negligent if she didn't make things better for everyone – a pattern learnt in childhood, a pattern that gave me power, but that also gave me an exhausting schedule. I wryly said to the doctor, 'You know, if I get worried I can see that I unconsciously calm myself down by helping others. On a bad day I'm in danger of rushing a whole Women's Guild of little old ladies to the other side of a road they never even wanted to cross!' I was given a homeopathic remedy that matched this type of compulsive overdoing. The view of a person who might benefit from this particular remedy is: 'The world is one great chaotic mess. The task of sorting it is impossible, but nonetheless that is my task – to impose a semblance of order over chaos. Although I lack the superhuman resources necessary, surrounding chaos upsets me so much that I must try to sort it out, single-handed if need be.' It wasn't hard to see the link between the remedy picture and my underlying energy state when stressed.

I also went for help to a Chinese herbalist who a friend had recommended. (I didn't take his herbal treatments until I had completed all chemotherapy since the two therapies might have interacted.) However, his view of the human body and the dynamic of its healing forces was hugely helpful to me. Conventional medical treatment for cancer largely seeks to eradicate the diseased cancerous cells in the body, giving the body the most toxic treatment it can bear in order to do so. While welcoming that, I also went for complementary treatments because I wished at the same time to do everything possible to enhance and support my body's own natural healing forces. I saw no contradiction whatsoever in this.

Treatment

When I described to the Chinese herbalist how apologetic I found I was feeling to my poor, tired body, to be putting it in front of such big and damaging guns as chemotherapy and radiotherapy, he replied with confidence. 'Oh, no, the body is the biggest gun.'

I realised the truth in his answer. Doctors can only give powerfully toxic treatments like chemotherapy and radiotherapy because our resilient body *is* the even-bigger gun. It can receive treatment so strong that the rapidly dividing cancer cells are killed. This same treatment also knocks the body's healthy cells on the head and yet, due to the body's remarkable healing power, the healthy cells slowly recover and life goes on.

Realising that the body was indeed the biggest gun changed my whole feeling about radiotherapy. The next day I swaggered down the angled corridor, and for the first time was able to look the machine above me in the eye as it clicked and zinged, delivering the radiation to my body. Through the help of a Chinese herbalist I no longer felt ambivalent about whether I was doing the right thing in having such aggressive treatment. I grinned at the radiotherapy machine with the zany thought, *I could fuse you if I wanted to*. I felt empowered, in charge of my decisions, and positive about having all the treatment available.

And then my mother died.

Mum

Following a series of hip and eye operations a few years previously, my Mum (widowed for over ten years) had reluctantly moved into sheltered housing near us in rural Scotland. She enjoyed seeing more of her grandchildren, but missed her roomy flat in Oxford. We settled into a regular routine of babysitting and shared outings that were full of laughter, but her underlying indignation at the whole ageing process often surfaced. She used to say to me, bursting with eighty-six-year-old exasperation, 'Don't ever get old, Mary. There is nothing to recommend it.' Mention of the alternative only raised her rancour, so I would simply change the subject (not always successfully).

Yet she was so much fun to be with once her mind was off her irritations. She was a remarkable woman who loved to travel and had adventured far and wide in her youth. Whenever family life got stressful she would forcefully say, 'If I hadn't got married, I was going to go to Hong Kong next ...' Another of her favourite sayings was, 'If I don't like my bed, I'll simply get up and remake it.'

The year before I developed cancer, something happened to her that could not be remade. After a bout of severe flu she became, and remained, very confused. When we had moved practice eighteen months previously she had needed to move into a nearby nursing home. I had hoped this would be for only a few months but her confusion deepened. She still knew us when we visited, but little else made much sense to her. The nursing home, run by nuns, was great. One nun said to me, as I commented on how easily Mum would do things for her but not for me, 'I think with your mother the veil goes a long way.' Mum had very happy memories of her time as a girl at a convent school, and in some ways she went back to that time now. I blessed the nuns who cared for her so well.

Mum would also have lucid moments. Before I had become ill I had suggested to her that we could look at buying a bigger house where we could all live together. She shook her head and said, 'It's never fair on the husband; and besides, the old person becomes a bit of a nonentity.' If there was one thing my Mum was not, and had no intention of becoming, it was a nonentity. When I once asked her how I could best help, she answered, 'Darling, I have become a little bit mad, and that's the hardest thing of all to help.' It was hard to see someone once so feisty now so confused. She developed an underlying exasperation with the whole blessed world for making so little sense to her. It was understandable but hard for her, and for others, to be with.

Yet the silver lining to her confusion was that once I became ill she remained happily unaware of it. Her normal self would have been sick with worry. The nursing home was a few miles away and I normally visited her on alternate days. I worried about her missing this when the operation prevented me from driving to visit her. When I asked her, three weeks after my operation, whether she had noticed that I had not been in for so long, she beamed and said, 'Do you know, darling, I hadn't.' It was such a relief to confirm that Mum had neither worried about me nor missed me.

Then, nearing the end of my month of radiotherapy, Mum suffered a major stroke. I rushed back from Edinburgh. One side of her body lay heavy and immobile in the bed. She looked at us with recognition yet was unable to talk. Over the next forty-eight hours the stroke progressed rapidly, and at a deep level I was relieved that it did. It felt time for my Mum to 'get away', as they say in Scotland; to leave the body that had become increasingly problematic and distressing to her. It was hard to watch Mum lie so still when she had always claimed she would defiantly 'remake her bed'. She developed a chest infection and I was with her when she died, peacefully, in the nursing home.

Mum's funeral was as grand as she would have wished it, held in the chapel at the nursing home. I was so grateful to the many friends who came, and to the nuns, staff and Mum's 'fellow inmates' (as she had always referred to them) who attended. Father MacLean took a full requiem Mass for her. I noticed the poor undertaker looking decidedly edgy as the service went on ... and on. After the Mass we were due to travel up to the crematorium in Edinburgh, and time slots there were tight. It became clear that the undertaker had been understandably unaware of the time required for a full requiem Mass and sign of peace amongst a benignly confused nursing home congregation. I found it lovely to receive so many smiles and handshakes – often several from the same person – from the folk around me, but it was the longest 'sign of peace' I have ever known. By the end the undertaker was looking ashen with worry. Eventually Mum's coffin was in the hearse and we all left the nursing home in a stately convoy, serenely waved off by the nuns. However, the minute we were out of the gates the undertaker put his foot down to make it to the crematorium on time. As my cousin Bernard later said, it was a case of 'Follow that hearse!'

After one of the fastest drives to Edinburgh I ever remember, we made it in time. I could just hear Mum indignantly saying, 'Well, *really*!' as we belted up the A68 and swerved round the corners. We were certainly not a solemn or ponderous funeral procession.

I have often wondered how hard that time must have been for my sister, standing at her mother's funeral alongside her only sister who had such a serious diagnosis. I simply felt hugely grateful to Donella for being there, for dealing with so much so well. And I felt a wave of gratitude to Mum for dying just then. She had been miserable and distressed since the dementia set in. Once she had the stroke it was as if she had decided 'Enough' and left. I felt her love was still with us, demonstrated even in the timing of her dying.

The funeral was a very close family time, but I was left numb and flat when the extended family dispersed. I dragged my way through the remaining three months of chemotherapy. I thought I would be delighted once I had completed all treatment. Instead I was listless and exhausted, uncertain whether all this could possibly have been worth it. John and I had booked a holiday to Madeira in February to celebrate Treatment End. I have chilly grey memories of the island in winter and of setting out on small excursions that rapidly ended in a taxi ride back to the hotel when I became too tired to continue.

It was simply a holiday too soon. My energy was very slow to return, but that summer we had one of our best family holidays ever. All four of us went on a sailing holiday to Greece. The sun shone on us, the children in their boats and we in ours. We all loved it. I vividly remember the elation of being far out in the bay on a windy day, sailing solo in my own small dinghy amid white waves and not capsizing, my heart singing.

Mum would have been delighted.

Optional Exercise (Four Minutes)
Imagination & Breathing

(Please move straight on to the next chapter if that feels right for you.)

For thirty seconds, imagine that you yourself have had to undergo an unwelcome operation. Nothing life-threatening, simply an operation that has changed your body in some way. Feel the sense of aversion, maybe even of despair or damage, of tiredness, as you surface from the anaesthetic and have to inhabit an altered 'you'. Allow every feeling all the space it needs, without arguing with it. See yourself looking at the scar on your abdomen or elsewhere, and experience the feelings that arise. Notice how your body being altered affects your sense of self, how your energy being lower affects your sense of confidence. Notice how you feel about the future in this moment. Hold all these feelings in an ocean of kindness so that, however painful, they can safely show themselves.

Now, in your imagination, switch to three months later, by which time you are fully healed.

For thirty seconds, imagine how you would feel to discover that your body has now fully adjusted to the changes. Your wound is barely noticeable. Your body is supple once again. You are back to normal functioning. You feel better than before the operation. You can hardly remember the strength of resistance you had at the time of the operation. Instead you feel empowered by your body's resilience and healing, more confident in your body and in yourself. Notice how you hold yourself, how you feel about possible challenges in the future, whether you feel more open, or more closed, about life in general.

Now for two minutes do this simple breathing exercise, breathing slowly in and out as follows:

On the in-breath: breathe in the sense of despair and dismay that you, or anyone else, can feel immediately after a body-altering operation.

On the out-breath: breathe out the joy that you, or anyone else, feels on discovering that the body is resilient and well able to fully heal, even from major trauma.

Remember:

In-breath: heaviness, dismay, despair (for yourself and others)

Out-breath: lightness, joy of healing, empowerment (for yourself and others)

Continue breathing in this way for two minutes, feeling the heaviness on the in-breath dissolving into lightness and going out to everyone on the out-breath. Allow the circle of people to widen to include yourself and as many others as is comfortable for you. Even strangers can be made welcome.

Final minute: Stop. Relax. Breathe normally and notice over the last minute how your body feels and how, in particular, your heart area feels.

We would maybe expect to feel burdened after taking in our own pain and that of others, yet all this dissolves into an out-breath that carries such lightness and healing that paradoxically many people find they feel more open, freer and lighter after this simple exercise.

Four

Finding a New Normal

Two months after the final course of chemotherapy I was impatient to get back to work as a part-time GP and put cancer and all its treatment firmly behind me. My blood tests had returned to normal. Compared to the greyness of chemotherapy I felt relatively well. It was definitely time to return to work, especially as I was noticing a nervousness beginning to build in me at the prospect of being the busy duty doctor once again. Time to just do it before I forgot how. I returned to work all set to be back to normal. I soon discovered I was not. My GP partners could not have been kinder, patients could not have been more welcoming, my hero-husband had taken over my night-time on call, yet I was deeply dismayed to find myself tired to my bones.

In part I could attribute this to the after-effects of the cytotoxic (literally, cell-poisoning) drugs, radiotherapy, and to the ongoing effect of tamoxifen, the anti-oestrogen drug I was to remain on for the next five years. The tumour cells in the biopsy had been tested and found to be hormone sensitive. I was grateful for this, since my chances of long-term survival would be improved by taking an anti-oestrogen tablet daily. With most natural oestrogens blocked, any tumour cells remaining in my body would be less likely to grow. However, the anti-oestrogen medication also meant that I now experienced a dramatic menopause. My periods stopped, my skin became drier, my moods brittle. This, together with ongoing exhaustion, made me feel like an old woman masquerading as a forty-five-year-old.

I reminded myself how awful it must be for even younger women, who perhaps had not had children, to have to take long-term anti-oestrogen treatment and feel this way. I would tell myself that my energy was returning every day (it wasn't), that I just needed to get more organised (I couldn't), that all GPs felt shattered on an on-call day (they did, but not like this) and that as long as I wore make-up my face looked quite healthy (debateable).

My lovely oncologist Dr Matheson had been so encouraging when I finished chemotherapy, brightly advising a good dose of retail therapy to celebrate. Finding this prescription infinitely preferable to all her previous ones, I complied. In bright new spring clothes, with a slap of rouge and lipstick, I felt quite chipper as I left for work each morning. A sense of 'Hey, look what I can go through and still come up smiling' buoyed me up for the first hour of each working day. Then tiredness would knock on the door. I'd tell myself that I wasn't really tired, just adjusting to being back at work again. That got me through the second hour. Then came a tiredness that didn't knock, that simply strode in and took over. I suddenly hit an invisible wall. Never have I been more grateful for the steaming mugs of tea left outside my door by receptionists who saw the exhaustion in my eyes. I would quietly sit and drink my tea, then feel able to see the extra emergency patients waiting. If I paced myself I could do it. I reminded myself of the many patients with cancer who are driven to go back to full-time work almost immediately after treatment in order to keep a job, in order to keep earning. This toxic combination of chronic ill health and acute money worries is borne by so many in today's society and stands in the way of their full recovery. I witnessed this daily in the practice as seriously ill patients on inadequate benefits struggled to make ends meet for themselves and their families. Present government austerity measures and changes to the benefit system continue to greatly worsen their plight, as is so brilliantly and tragically portrayed in the 2016 film *I, Daniel Blake*.

I was lucky as a doctor to be among those better off, but I still had to find out whether or not I could do the job I had done before. I had my doubts; I sense all returnees must have them too. Maybe I was no longer fit for such demanding work. But by now I had been off sick for a full eleven months. My GP partners had been nothing but supportive, telling me to take as long as I needed. But as a partner myself, I knew the huge strain just one absent partner creates within a practice. However generously the other partners carry the extra load, the work strain is cumulative as the months go on. Two months after completing all treatment, I had to return and simply find out whether I could do the job or not. I had always enjoyed my work and hoped to settle back fairly easily into such a good team.

Once back I was shocked, and a little frightened, to find that I had so little energy in my tank. A GP day is varied, stimulating and unpredictable. You never know what is going to happen next when your practice cares for over seven thousand patients. The interruptions and unexpected emergencies come when they will, not when you timetable them. When you are the doctor on-call for that day's emergencies, you go into work feeling rather like an athlete on the starting blocks without knowing in which direction, or how fast, you will be asked to run. You sincerely hope that you won't be required to run in too many different directions at the same time. Going back to work after chemotherapy, I realised I felt more like an eighty-year-old on the starting blocks. I felt neither quick-witted nor quick-bodied. Alarmed for patient safety, for the first few months I did routine surgeries but employed a locum doctor to do my emergency visits. I was determined I wasn't going to put any patient at risk while I put this new, frail me back into the workplace and through her paces.

I shared the sentiments of one eighty-year-old patient who came into the consulting room looking so spry in her make-up and Jacques Vert suit that I just had to tell her how good she looked. She raised one eyebrow as she sat down and said drily, 'Aye, doctor, the wheel's spinning but the hamster's dead.'

I was tired, but also confused. I had no idea what my body was up to. I didn't know whether the cancer had been eliminated or not, and taking tamoxifen threw in the further confounding factor of unpredictable menopausal symptoms. The resulting hot flushes were both frequent and relentless, disturbing sleep as bedclothes were flung on and off. As a GP I had always (or so I thought) been sympathetic to the many menopausal women who came to me complaining vociferously about hot flushes. However, inwardly I used to quietly think, 'But surely it's only being a bit hot. Is that really such an overwhelming symptom?' Yup, under a veneer of female solidarity, some young women GPs can be less sympathetic than their male counterparts towards menopausal women.

Well now I knew the baking heat of their discontent – I was standing in their sweat-filled, sleep-deprived moccasins. For a few random minutes, as your brain seems to melt, the heat is so commanding that all you can do is simply wait, normal functioning temporarily out. You broadcast your state to all and sundry by turning briefly but unmissably beetroot. Within seconds, beads of sweat form on your forehead, join into rivulets and drip into your eyes. The rest of your body rapidly follows suit. You imagine a pool of perspiration the size of Loch Lomond forming around your feet but dare not look. Then suddenly the switch is off, your brain comes back online and normal services are resumed ... until the next time. I defy any man to keep his cool were his body to play such unexpected tricks on him 24/7.

Women who find hot flushes overwhelming and ongoing are frequently treated with Hormone Replacement Therapy (HRT), since oestrogen replacement resolves these symptoms instantly. Forbidden all oestrogen myself, I had to struggle on through all the temperature changes my body could throw at me while silently envying the patients to whom I could hand out HRT prescriptions. They looked so calm, collected and youthful when they returned to pick up another script, brightly saying, 'HRT just makes me feel like myself again.' My delight for them was clouded by sadness for myself. Calm, collected, bright and 'myself' summed up everything I was not. And yet it is remarkable what the body adjusts to and tolerates. It is equally remarkable what patients adjust to and tolerate in their doctor. Patients seemed not to mind as the calm, attentively listening GP in front of them suddenly morphed into a demented, garment-shedding flurry, jumper over head, earrings flying in all directions. Male patients kindly carried on as if nothing was happening. Older female patients grinned sympathetically, commenting, 'Hot flush, huh?' I realised it was time to rethink the work clothes. I dropped the earrings – I'd lost half of them anyway – and took to wearing cardigans.

However, my unease and discontent ran far deeper than just my menopausal symptoms. I had expected to feel elated to have finished all treatment and be back at work. Instead I felt exhausted and more deeply unsure than I'd ever felt in my life – unsure whether my brain was still sharp enough to give good medical care to my patients, and even less sure that my body was well enough. Finishing an intense course of chemotherapy and radiotherapy is a weird anti-climax. I had been counting off the treatments one by one, my only aim being to complete the course and get back to normal life. It was such a relief to tick off that last treatment and wave goodbye to nausea, but to my surprise it began to feel eerie not to be going back for more.

During treatment my body had felt like a battleground and I had accepted that. I understood the necessity for pushing treatment hard. If there was a chance of a permanent cure, who in their right mind wouldn't go for that? The cancer specialists aim to give the maximum amount of chemotherapy and radiotherapy that your body can tolerate; the dose that will kill off any remaining cancer cells while allowing healthy cells to recover. Too low a dose and the cancer cells are not killed. Too high a dose and your healthy cells do not recover. Cancer patients and their doctors ride this razor edge of not too much, but not too little, treatment.

There's definitely a buzz of battle during chemotherapy. You know exactly what you and your doctors are doing, your body taking the poison each time and then recovering. The doctors and nurses are attentive and alert for every side effect or problem. Everyone knows what you are going through and is there to help you in every way possible. Red Cross style parcels from friends just keep on coming, and you feel grateful for every one of them. You feel shattered, but also reassured that with the treatment you are courageously doing everything possible to reduce the risk of any future cancer recurrence. And you feel that you have a brilliant team supporting you every time you go 'over the top' and take another dose of chemo or radiotherapy. Although you dread the nausea every time, you begin to know how to deal with it. You accustom yourself.

Unilateral ceasefire

And then, on a certain date, all that fierce treatment stops. The silence is surprising. Suddenly, medical high command has called 'Enough' and declared that the ongoing barrage, the shelling of the cancer, is over – Treatment End, the moment you have been longing for. Initially you are delighted and bask in the knowledge of your remarkable body and all the strong treatment it has been able to withstand. But as time passes it is impossible not to wonder, *If my healthy cells have been able to recover each time, what if some of the cancer cells have recovered too?*

You begin to realise that it is a unilateral ceasefire that has been called. You feel like asking your medical team, 'Did you consult the other side about this? Did the cancer cells agree to this ceasefire as well?' You wonder whether all that toxic ammunition directed at any remaining cancer cells was indeed enough to kill them. Awake in the middle of the night, you catastrophise and question whether a few cancer cells might just be playing dead for now, only to surface later. You wonder whether the enemy trenches really are empty, as claimed. Now begins the period – hopefully a very long one – of waiting to find out whether the treatment was successful ... or not.

I read somewhere that some cancer patients find this initial post-treatment period akin to having fallen asleep in a hotel room, only to be woken by a thud as the shoe of the drunken, sleeping guest in the room above falls off and lands on the bedroom floor. Much as they want to, the person in the room beneath cannot go back to sleep, as they wait for that other shoe to fall off. That state of being semi-alert, yet wanting to forget and relax, perfectly matched my own uneasy sense of waiting and wondering.

I needed help to deal with this state of inner watchfulness, a waiting for that which I most dreaded. I sense all cancer patients experience this in their own individual way. I was grateful when friends beamed and told me how well I looked. I would nod, agree and beam back, while silently wondering, *But am I truly well, and if so – for how long?* And the answer is: you simply do not know. You look at your family, and your family looks at you, the same unasked and unanswerable question in both sets of eyes. You ask the doctors, and they don't know either. They can only give you statistics for your type of cancer as a general guide. In many forms of cancer, total cure rates are now very high. However, back then, with the aggressive type of cancer I had, treatment was still evolving. I was given no 'cure rate'. Only the overall statistic: forty per cent of patients still alive at five years (many already with a recurrence), sixty per cent dead within five years, even after all that treatment. I wished I'd never asked.

The patient in front of you was not in the trial

Evidence for different types of cancer and their treatment is now good. Survival rates for the type of cancer I had in 1997 have improved markedly in the past twenty years. Also, many cancers are now curable. If you are reading this and have cancer, and doctors have told you that your type of cancer is 100 per cent curable, simply take the full treatment, celebrate the fact such treatment is both available and curative, and return to normal life expectancy without any worries of a recurrence.

What I write next refers only to myself and to fellow patients whose type of cancer does not, as yet, have a certain cure. Although the statistics that doctors give refer only to patients with your particular type of disease, these statistics always and only refer to a group of patients in the past. They are a record of how the disease grew or remitted in a group of patients who lived years ago, a group of which you are not part. The statistics for the group of patients you *are* part of do not yet exist, have not yet been gathered. You will form part of those statistics, you are in each moment forming part of them, but you have no way of knowing which part of them you will fall into. Will it be the long-term survivor group, the short-term survivor group or somewhere in between? All you know is that you will be somewhere in one of those three groups. Statistics can never predict how the future for you – unique, quirky you, the individual who has this illness – will unfold.

This was personal uncertainty of an order I had never known before. Worse, there was no resolving it. Such ongoing uncertainty about future health and longevity is part and parcel of the diagnosis of any aggressive form of cancer. I came to realise that I was out at sea: the storm of treatment might have died down, the water was now calmer, but a return to the safe shore of assuredly healthy ground was not possible. I realised I could never make land and return to that carefree past when I didn't have cancer. And I hadn't a clue about the quality of the boat I was in, still less how to sail it. And the winds were strong – the equally strong opposing winds of hope (fervent, that I would now remain well) and fear (desperate, that I would not). You can busy yourself, distract yourself, fling yourself into good works, have excessive fun – I did all four and more – but the undertow of alarmed not-knowing is always there, always pulling.

I needed help to find a way of living with this. I sensed that all the therapeutic 'fix-it' avenues (counselling and massage, homeopathy, Chinese herbalism, acupuncture) I had already travelled could not answer this one. What if, despite all the 'putting-right' of this or that imbalance in my body or psyche, things still went seriously wrong? I desperately needed to discover how to live steadily in the face of all possibilities, including the possibility of my dying soon of this cancer. Otherwise I would never know peace again.

Five

A Wider Way of Seeing

I think that when you are ill, you in the West suffer
much more than we do. In Tibet, as soon as we are born
we know that suffering, illness and death are a part of life.
To some they come early ... to some late.

This response from Lama Yeshe took me by surprise. I had
just described to him all that had happened to me over the
past year: the sudden diagnosis of an aggressive cancer, the
exhausting treatment, the ongoing uncertainty regarding
my health and energy, and my mother's recent death. Most
of my friends were shocked and concerned for our family. I
was pretty shocked and concerned myself. One of the nurses
who cared for my mum after her stroke had said to me, as
I arrived from another week of radiotherapy in Edinburgh,
'Sure, you're not needing to go looking for your worries
just now, are you Mary?' I could only agree. Yet here was
Lama Yeshe, Abbot of Samye Ling Tibetan Buddhist monastery (Eskdalemuir, Scotland), to whom I had just recounted
all my troubles, sitting calm and unperturbed. It was as if I

had just told my story to a mountain. He was so seemingly unmoved that part of me wanted to lean forward, tap his arm and ask, 'And did you get the bit about my mother?'

Lama Yeshe's response was different from everyone else's, my own included. I had reacted with alarm and distress to a cancer diagnosis in my forties. I was acutely concerned for my children while still grieving deeply for my own much loved mother. I had come to view myself as particularly unlucky, even abnormally so. Repeated calamity causes one to become rather self-absorbed. Or maybe self-absorption leads one to interpret events as calamitous? Either way, my sense was simply that everything had been going fine, and now everything was very far from fine and could not readily be made fine again. 'Why me?' wasn't really my question since 'Why not me?' seemed equally valid.

It was more that I couldn't shift an underlying sense of shocked recoil and horror at my cancer diagnosis, Mum's dementia, stroke and death, and – possibly soon – my own death. With two young children, what was there to be calm about in that lot? Yet here was someone who listened fully and whose calm remained unruffled. 'Frightened/needy me' could have interpreted this as indifference – yet it so clearly was not. After I had spoken he simply told me that nothing abnormal had happened, that sickness and death were a normal part of life, that they come 'to some early, to some late' and that failure to recognise and accept these simple facts causes us a lot of extra suffering. We only talked for a few minutes more. There truly was little more to say. I came out from Lama Yeshe's room dazed, surprised, not really knowing what I was feeling.

Part of my mind wanted to argue with him and say, 'But this is big, this feels too much.' Yet how can you possibly say that to someone who I knew had lost his country, his monastery, his family and the majority of his travelling companions when escaping from Tibet in 1959? Out of a group of three hundred Tibetans fleeing the Chinese that year, only thirteen made it through to India. The others were caught or shot by the Chinese, or died on the journey from sickness, hypothermia and hunger. Lama Yeshe was only fifteen when he and his two brothers finally arrived in India. Like so many Tibetans, they then contracted tuberculosis in the refugee camps. One brother died from it. Lama Yeshe had a lung removed but recovered.

How was it that Lama Yeshe, having suffered so much, was now completely calm, happy, at ease, and available to see anyone who asked to see him? I was not a Buddhist, had not needed to be – anyone at all could ask to see him, and this was my first meeting with him. He had made no mention of religion, had not attempted to give me any new view involving a single afterlife or reincarnation. How was it then that, despite my own inner shakiness and alarm, he had been able to effortlessly and totally transmit a sense that all I had experienced was simply a normal part of life, not that remarkable, simply to be accepted and got on with?

As I drove away from the monastery one part of my brain was saying, *Well, that wasn't very sympathetic, was it?* However, another part of me, a part that maybe I hadn't consulted or contacted yet, was undeniably feeling strangely at ease. I felt so surprised, yet okay, that I stopped the car and went for a walk by the river. I asked myself, *So what are you really feeling now, after that meeting?*

To my astonishment I realised that, for the first time in a year, I was feeling normal. The anxiety, dread and frantic search for answers within me – the tension that had risen to such a high degree – had dramatically slackened off. Nothing had changed in terms of my diagnosis and prognosis, yet everything had changed in terms of how I looked at it all. The whole situation now felt workable (and has remained so).

I have recounted that conversation on many occasions since. Folk divide into those who immediately get it and grin, and those who look very shocked indeed that anyone could react so seemingly unsympathetically to such a story. To the second group I always say, 'But if you had been there, being spoken to by Lama Yeshe yourself, truly you would have absorbed his message too.' He was not unsympathetic; he was open and kind – but he was also completely honest and quite unprepared to collude with anyone's proffered sense of being wronged or hard done by. I had asked to see him because I had attended a few courses at Samye Ling monastery in previous years and been impressed by the people giving them. I sensed that there was help and a wider view here and I had come looking for strength, any strength, as my own supplies felt perilously close to empty. I had asked for help, been given an appointment, had not been asked to go along with any belief-set. I simply met strength, steadiness, and the true compassion of telling the straightforward truth – all embodied in Lama Yeshe.

My mind did not know what to do with any of this but somehow, without many words, a quiet steadiness within me was revived on encountering such massive steadiness in him. My gaze widened and I saw that of course sickness, old age and death are a normal part of life. There was no fault involved, no mistake to correct. There was simply some suffering and tenderness to feel. All tension left as I realised this. Sadness remained that Mum had died, that I had got cancer. But from that time on, my crazy argument against it all stilled. Of course I still keenly hoped that the cancer would now stay away, but my desperate desire to be certain of cure disappeared, never to return again. Something in the shift in my perception that happened then, when I was desperate, has stayed and grown ever since.

I would love to write that the tiredness also wore off and full energy returned, as I have seen it return in many patients after intensive cancer treatment. Although my fatigue eased considerably over that first year of recovery, my physical energy never bobbed back to what it had been before. For some patients it's just like that. Initially I was so impatient to 'keep on getting better' that I pushed myself to follow the family up hills, to join friends on long walks. Despite returning exhausted and wiped out for the next day, I kept pushing, imagining I only needed to build up fitness again. I was so happy to be alive, surely I just needed to man-up on this one, climb the hills, and more energy would come? As they say in Glasgow: 'It's the bloody hope that gets you every time.'

I am a fine one to be writing a book about acceptance. It seems I come to consider acceptance only once all possible attempts to alter and bargain with the situation have utterly failed. Maybe that is so for most of us. As Elisabeth Kübler-Ross wrote about the stages of grief (denial, bargaining, anger, depression, acceptance), these are just the feelings we all seem to move through on our way to accepting an unwelcome reality. Once I simply accepted my energy levels as they were – much lower than before, but good enough – peace broke out. The struggle had been in longingly looking for more. I couldn't feel too sad about low energy; I was so relieved to be a survivor, experiencing no actual cancer symptoms. I explained to my family, 'I'm fine, it's just that my energy levels seem to have moved ten years on – they're more those of a fifty-five-year-old than a forty-five-year-old.'

I was fortunate to have a job that was part-time and wasn't too physical. Over the following years I continued to work as a family doctor and care for patients with many illnesses at all stages, including cancer. I understood the nature of this illness, and was always keenly aware that simply in surviving I was a lot luckier than many fellow patients of my age and younger. Although I now had a much deeper understanding of what it was like to be diagnosed with a life-threatening illness, I made sure I never said to a patient in similar circumstances, 'I know how you feel', simply because I knew I didn't know how they felt. Another person can never know just how a given diagnosis is hitting someone else. I tended to keep quiet about my own story so as not to get in the way of theirs. I'm keenly aware of the same risk in writing this book. Every patient with cancer or any other diagnosis is utterly unique. Each person's experience is valid only for them. Reading too vivid an account of a fellow patient's journey can inspire, but can also daunt and depress.

My sole purpose in writing this book follows the guidance given to me by Lama Yeshe: 'Write about how you were when full of fear about the cancer, and how you are without that fear. Write about how you somehow found a way not to suffer, and how not to make your family suffer. Write only with the intention of helping others and their families to suffer less.'

Six

Recurrence, 2010

A cold winter we had of it in 2009. The coldest winter in Britain for over thirty years. Snow started to fall softly mid-December and forgot to stop. Snowploughs cleared the way for families to somehow reach each other in time for Christmas. After the necessary festive overeating we went for long hill walks, our springer spaniel Tess leaping through the deep drifts like an alongside porpoise. Heavy snow covered the hills, blanketing out the noise of the world. It was a lovely family time together. It had all been so easy, yet I found myself exhausted as I packed the decorations away for another year. With everyone now gone and John busy back at work, I wasn't surprised to feel a bit flat as I vacuumed the pine needles. I was sure thousands of fellow vacuum-wielders were feeling similarly listless and wan. Yet it was odd to find myself quite *this* tired.

I was still adjusting to retirement from general practice eighteen months earlier. I found I really missed the contact with both patients and practice partners. Days at work had been demanding, but always interesting. As one colleague

75

described it, a GP's job is 'to sort the unsortable' in impossibly short, ten-minute appointment slots. You go home each night checking whether you've missed anything. It is a challenging, enjoyable, but often troubling job. As John would say, so unreassuringly, 'You're only as good as your last diagnosis.'

In 2008 I had started to feel I wasn't on top of my game any more. I worried increasingly that I wasn't keeping up to date with the latest medical journals, I was taking longer to get through my list of home visits and I was coming home later and later in the evenings, trying to complete the paperwork. I think most GPs would recognise themselves in this listing of burdens. But my worry was that I might start to miss things; that patients could suffer if I clung on to my job while not feeling up to it. My heart goes out to young doctors, and all young workers today, who will be expected to keep going at the workface long into their sixties. As a GP at fifty-six my exhaustion at the end of each working day was almost total. Driving home at 8pm one night, I remember thinking, *I'm almost too tired to breathe – mustn't forget to do that.* It was time to stop.

I had expected a new lease of energy after dropping the day job. However, the happily anticipated surge of *chi* (life force) failed to materialise. Eighteen months into retirement I was listless and unsure where to direct the little energy I had. I had been to my excellent GP: routine medical tests and even a cardiology check proved clear, my coronary arteries unaffected by the radiotherapy thirteen years before. We left the investigations at that, vague tiredness and mild melancholia being my only complaints. Maybe it was all just retirement blues. No one, including myself, suggested a

CT scan as I had no weight loss or any symptoms suggestive of a cancer recurrence. Besides, the breast cancer had been so long ago.

Which was why I told myself not to be dramatic when, early in January 2010, my eye was caught by a small swelling just beside my sternum. Funny how the corner of our eye picks up even the slightest change in something as familiar as our own body. I didn't think I had seen the swelling before. Was it new? It was only just noticeable: a tiny, innocent looking bulge in the flesh beside my breastbone, nestling between my third and fourth ribs. I felt it and it was soft, nothing like the hard nodule I had felt in my breast in 1997. John and I both thought it was probably a benign fluid-filled cyst. Yet it was on the left, the side the cancer had been on. Somehow, just like the first time, I sensed that this might be serious. Strange to be suddenly alert to the possibility of recurrence after years of being carefree. My GP sent me for an ultrasound scan.

A day at the hospital

I hoped the ultrasound would confirm the lump to be a cyst, but John and I were wary. We went to the appointment together. The radiologist eyed his screen in silence. I waited for a reassurance that never came. After repeating the test he said, 'I'm afraid it's not a cyst. It appears to be solid.' Suddenly I was afraid. This was now a cancer recurrence until proved otherwise. It was so hard to believe that thirteen healthy years after all the breast cancer treatment in 1997, this soft swelling might be the first sign of its return.

My ultrasound appointment extended into a rapidly arranged CT scan with an appointment to see the surgeon afterwards, the same reassuringly straightforward man who had performed my mastectomy thirteen years previously. I knew at once that the scan results must be serious – the surgeon looked so very unhappy as he invited John and me into his consulting room. He seemed genuinely shocked. I was, after all, perfectly well, just tired. He told us that the tiny lump I had found was the visible part of a much larger mass inside my chest. Its outline was irregular. It was likely to be cancer, probably a recurrence of my long-ago breast cancer, this time in one of the lymph nodes behind the sternum. He said it was extraordinary that a mass this large was causing no symptoms. A biopsy would be necessary. I asked the surgeon how big the whole mass actually was. He made a rapid gesture with his hand indicating a lump roughly the size of a small lemon. I was shocked. In fact he was being kind. I later learned from the radiologist that the CT scan showed a mass behind my sternum that was ten centimetres in diameter – more the size of a grapefruit.

John and I returned home pole-axed. We deeply appreciated how speedily further tests had been done, we had nodded and asked all the right questions at all the right times, but it was only once we were home that the immensity of the bad news really sank in. Of course, as doctors we had always known that cancer can recur decades later, but thirteen years of good health had begun to seem like quite a secure stretch of clear water between me and cancer. I had been at a bit of a loose end after retiring from work, wondering what I would do next. I never imagined it would be this. We had just enjoyed an energetic family Christmas; my only symptom was tiredness. A chest mass ten centimetres in diameter, showing up now? Surely not.

How rapidly our lives can change.

I remembered the deal I'd made with the universe when the cancer first came in 1997: *Just let the kids grow up without losing their mum. Please just allow that and I'll be happy.* Adam and Rebecca were now twenty-four and twenty-one. The universe had kept its side of the deal, but now I wanted to renegotiate: surely I was too fit and well for this set of results? However, the biopsy later that week confirmed the surgeon's prediction. This mass was indeed a recurrence of the original breast cancer. My heart sank at the prospect of more chemo or radiotherapy. Both had been worth doing when the family was young, when the chances of cure were there. But both treatments had exhausted me then. Now, aged fifty-seven, already tired, with a large recurrence that I couldn't imagine would be curable, I sagged at the thought of further aggressive treatment.

Treatment options

The next week we met Dr Carolyn Bedi, a young and highly competent oncologist, to discuss treatment options. If I had been asked to list the qualities I would have wanted in an oncologist, she had them all in spades: she was warm, sympathetic, well informed, and quietly and skilfully direct in communicating all necessary information while giving us space to adjust and discuss. I felt I was in competent hands.

What to do with such a mass? Dr Bedi told me that my case had been discussed at the weekly oncology meeting with the surgeons. She told us that current treatment options were surgical removal, radiotherapy and hormone treatment. I was relieved chemotherapy was not recommended, since the mass was local and I was presently well. I was amazed to learn that the surgeons had offered to remove this mass. It was so central, impinging on all the major thoroughfares that course through the chest. It was close to, or pressing against, major arteries and veins as well as the heart, vital nerves, glands, and probably my gullet and airways too. Who in their right mind would want to go wielding a scalpel in amongst that lot?

The surgeons also advised that any operation would involve the removal of my breastbone (sternum), replacing it with an artificial sternum made of titanium. This I had never heard of. How would my ribs attach to *that*? I felt we were slipping into the fantastic. I said I could only imagine undergoing such an extensive and risky operation if there was some chance of a cure. When closely questioned, the surgeons said that the operation would be 'heroic but non-curative'. I was surprised they even offered such an operation. However, I realised that they looked at my CT scan with surgical eyes. They saw how close this mass was to vital structures, how serious my prognosis was, and therefore they offered me the best chance from their point of view – surgical removal of this threatening mass that was only going to grow further. I was not ungrateful, but nor was I drawn to say yes.

Another option was radiotherapy. I asked, 'But didn't that area have maximum radiotherapy thirteen years ago?' Dr Bedi agreed that it had, but she thought we could get away with a limited five-day course of repeat radiotherapy to this area. However, she added that since the mass was so large, the dose of radiotherapy given would have to be large too, and would once again irradiate my heart. So there were also serious risks with radiotherapy. The other treatment recommended was anti-oestrogen hormone therapy, since the biopsy had shown that the tumour was hormone-sensitive.

To me the answer was clear. If I went for the 'heroic' surgery I might well die on the operating table or soon after, and could remain a long-term intensive care patient even if the unbelievable bodily rearrangements that the surgeons were proposing went well. Any convalescence would certainly be protracted. I saw no point in putting myself, my family, or indeed the surgeons, nurses and the NHS, through all that when the gain could well be so short-lived – literally. Radiotherapy was similarly unappealing, since the dose had to match the largesse of the mass. I could remember how wiped-out I had felt after radiotherapy the first time round. I decided that since I was well for now, the only treatment that seemed appropriate was anti-oestrogen hormone treatment. I told Dr Bedi that I would also seek treatment from a friend in India who was an excellent homeopathic physician.

She nodded in understanding at my decision, gave me a prescription for the anti-oestrogen tablets but looked concerned as we parted, saying, 'The problem is that you may well run into complications from this mass before these gentler treatments have a chance to act.' I, in turn, nodded in understanding.

That evening
After a very quiet supper that evening, John asked me what I wanted to do. What *did* I want to do? To my surprise, I knew. Before Christmas I had read a book about Alice Herz Sommer, a Czech pianist who as a young mother had

survived Theresienstadt concentration camp during the Second World War. A friend had recently given me a DVD of a moving documentary film about Herz Sommer, [1] who was now over one hundred years old. I wanted to soak up wisdom from this remarkable survivor.

So that bizarre evening we watched Alice Herz Sommer play the piano with her gnarled fingers. We heard her recount details of her extraordinary life. She was born and brought up in bohemian Prague between the wars, her happy childhood filled with music and culture. Then came the German invasion. First her mother was taken to the camps. The order for Alice to follow came soon after. Regarding the horrors she saw in the concentration camp, she said, 'I did not talk of them after the war, and I will not talk of them now.' Instead she spoke of the way music saved her then, and still saved her now, adding, 'I am Jewish, but Beethoven is my religion.' She spoke of her joy when playing the piano for fellow inmates in the camp: 'Whenever I knew that I had a concert, I was happy that day. Music is magic. We performed in the council hall before an audience of a hundred-and-fifty hopeless, sick and hungry people. They lived for music. It was like food for them.'

Although her husband died in Dachau concentration camp shortly before liberation, she spoke only of how he had saved her life, and the life of their son, through his wise advice to her before he was taken away. Although, by the time the film was made, she had already outlived her only and precious son, who died suddenly in his sixties, she repeated many times throughout the film how fortunate she had been to have such a good son, and how fortunate she was now to be visited by her wonderful grandson. She said that optimism – looking at the good in life rather than at the bad – was the key to her life.

This film about her wisdom and fortitude was about the only thing John and I could both have watched that evening. Even at over one hundred years old, Alice Herz Sommer made a lasting impression with her gentle piano playing, her quiet dignity despite all she had weathered, her reticence about past horrors and her ongoing appreciation for all the gifts in her life. Something struck me about the strength with which she chose where she placed her attention. I realised that, even in my situation – maybe especially in my situation – I could follow her lead. I, too, could choose where I put my attention, what I dwelt on and what I did not dwell on. I am so grateful to her for surviving, for staying optimistic despite the horror that surrounded her – for staying sensitive to beauty. She helped me to see that my present situation, though shockingly sudden and stark, need not absorb and command my whole attention. The world was still both beautiful and terrible, even if my cancer had returned. It was up to me now where I placed my attention, up to me what decisions I made, up to me how I lived my remaining life. That evening, the remarkable Alice Herz Sommer helped both John and me to lift and focus our gaze once again.

The next day I emailed Dr Rajan Sankaran in Mumbai.

Seven

A Skype Call to Mumbai

Before I describe my 2010 Skype consultation with Dr Rajan Sankaran – homeopathic doctor, teacher and friend – I must break off from my story as a cancer patient and briefly describe my journey as a newly qualified doctor in the 1970s.

I was very firm in my opinions way back then. As a young doctor I had heard of homeopathy but never found it appealing. If anything, I was a bit impatient with people who used it. How could they believe in a homeopathic remedy having an effect when the original substance, be it animal vegetable or mineral, had been diluted one-in-a-hundred times so many times that there was little chance of the eventual remedy even containing a single molecule of the original substance? The logical medical student in me had been taught that drugs acted by a molecule of that drug linking with a receptor site in the body and causing a certain effect. Regarding homeopathy, I took the patronising stance of 'at least these remedies do no harm' and concluded that they could only have an effect … on gullible minds.

Then, two years after graduating, I spent three months in a Camphill Community, a residential school for children in need of special care, near Aberdeen. My views about complementary therapies – and also about community living – slowly began to open up. I so admired the staff there. I helped in the aphasic class and watched how the young teachers interacted warmly, patiently with children who could not speak. I was also a dormitory parent. This meant that each morning I gently woke three boys who shared a small dormitory, helped them get ready for the day, and then helped them get to bed in the evening. One of the three was a highly intelligent ten-year-old boy called Simon. He'd had a wretched childhood and had deep emotional problems. He was almost impossible to get up in the morning and over the weeks my morning mood became less and less gentle. In despair I said to the wonderful Camphill doctor, Thomas Weihs, 'I don't know what to do with Simon. I can practically turn the bed upside down in the morning and he still won't get up. And he's so mean to the other boys.' Dr Weihs looked thoughtful. 'Yes,' he said gently, 'I can understand that. It can't be easy to get up and be Simon every day.' That changed everything for me. Suddenly I saw from Simon's point of view how desperately painful his life had been, how little he wanted any of it. Why should he want to get up to another day? My impatience disappeared – and Simon started getting up in the morning. Music therapy was also used with wonderful effect at Camphill. They used homeopathic remedies too, and clearly trusted them. My prejudice stood down slightly.

Later, in Africa, I saw all too clearly the limits of what John and I could and could not do. I became less high-handed regarding the supreme authority of conventional medicine. We got to know the local *singanga* (traditional healer), a courteous, elderly man, intriguingly named Mr Paison. He started referring patients he knew we could help, and we noticed how well those suffering with psychological problems did in his care. We were very grateful for this since Malawi had only one psychiatric hospital for the whole country and the only drug for psychiatric problems in our entire hospital pharmacy was chlorpromazine (one of the early drugs used in psychotic illness). My mind opened a shade more to all that I did not know.

In the 1980s I resumed work as a part time GP in rural Scotland. You get to know your patients very well as a GP in a small community. You see them over many years. You especially get to know those patients who are seriously unwell and who are not getting better. You know them, you know their families, you see the effects that chronic illness has on the whole family − on children, spouses, siblings and parents. As the local GP you know just how much the whole family is suffering.

Two such chronically ill patients came to see me regularly. (As in all cases where patients are referred to in this book, names and details have been altered to protect patient anonymity.)

Brenda

Brenda was thirty years old, married, with a fourteen-year-old son. She suffered from aggressive inflammatory bowel disease. I had never seen bowel disease this aggressive. Ten years previously she'd had an acute flare-up and had to have a large part of her bowel removed; the surgeons had managed to avoid a colostomy. Since then she had had many flare-ups, which had slowly settled on steroids and auto-immune therapy. However, over the past year she had had a flare-up that was not settling. Her gastroenterologist increased the steroid to a very high daily dose while keeping her auto-immune therapy at maximum. Her bowel was so diseased and inflamed, her life so miserable, that surgical removal of most of her remaining bowel was being considered. She was heading for an ileostomy (an opening on her abdomen that would allow her small bowel to empty into an external plastic pouch). She desperately wanted to avoid this as she would then be wearing a bag for the rest of her life.

She asked me if there was no other treatment we could try first. In desperation – and only because the conventional therapeutic cupboard was bare – I said that as a last resort we could refer her to the Glasgow Homeopathic Hospital, adding that I thought she would probably be operated on before she could be seen there. But she was insistent so I wrote a letter of referral explaining the urgency of Brenda's current situation. I glanced through her extensive notes, checking that I had not missed anything from her past history. Hidden at the back I found a letter from the obstetrician at Raigmore Hospital, Inverness, from fourteen years ago, when her son had been born. Brenda had never referred to this time and the letter was just one among hundreds in her file. I learned that Brenda had become pregnant aged 16, unmarried and coming from a religious family living in a tightly conservative community in the Highlands. She successfully concealed her pregnancy from her family, perhaps even from herself. The shock of her going into early labour at home, far from medical help in an isolated area, must have been overwhelming for the teenager, and indeed for her whole family.

The ambulance was called but her premature baby was born just before it arrived. The baby cried heartily and was kept warm. Then Brenda started haemorrhaging. She was rushed along winding, single-track roads in a blue-light ambulance, a journey of ninety minutes, to the nearest hospital. She nearly died on the way from blood loss. She reached hospital just in time, was operated on and given extensive blood transfusions. The baby's biological father was never named. Her family helped her care for the baby and she later married another man, who adopted her son as his own.

No wonder Brenda had never mentioned such a traumatic time. Yet all past history is significant, and I communicated the full details of this episode, and the fact that Brenda had never referred to it, to the homeopathic doctor in Glasgow. He saw her the following week and prescribed the remedy Staphysagria at 200C potency (yes, that same high dilution that I knew contained not a molecule of the original substance). Brenda took the remedy – a mere three tablets over just one day – and I expected nothing.

The results were astonishing. Symptoms eased immediately and within two weeks her bloody diarrhoea (ongoing for a year) had stopped. We tentatively started reducing her steroids. Over the next two months her prednisolone was reduced from 40mg a day to 5mg a day and she remained well. Soon she was on only 2mg a day. She said she had never felt better.

I didn't know what to make of it all. I spoke with the other doctors looking after her and we all agreed the change had happened only after the homeopathic remedy. I had to take notice of that, yet the sceptic in me was still doubtful. Then, over a year later, Brenda had a mild flare-up of her stomach problems. I suggested she repeat the homeopathic remedy and was surprised to find her very reluctant to do so.

I said, 'Brenda, but it's only a homeopathic remedy, and it seemed to get you better last time you took it.'

She answered, 'I know it got my stomach better. It's something else. I've never told anyone this – I thought you'd think I was going mad. When I took those three homeopathy tablets a year ago, that night I relived that journey in the ambulance fourteen years ago. I bled and nearly died after my baby was born up north. I'd forgotten all about that time and it was terrifying to relive it all again – all that blood. I don't want to repeat those tablets if those memories might come back again.'

I phoned the doctor at the homeopathic hospital. He didn't sound surprised. He explained that Staphysagria is a remedy indicated for deep suppression of past trauma. The homeopathic view takes everything into the picture: all physical *and* emotional symptoms over time. Everything about the person is relevant to the choice of remedy. According to this view, severe emotional suppression can lead to later physical symptoms, as in Brenda's case. The homeopathic doctor explained that Brenda's reliving of her past trauma, after taking the Staphysagria 200C, was a one-off – a clearing-out from her emotional system of a memory that had been deeply denied and therefore strongly held in her body. He told me to assure Brenda that she would not have such a vivid playback on retaking the remedy now. Brenda seemed happy with this and repeated the remedy with no subsequent emotional disturbance. Her stomach problems eased once again. Ten years on, she remained well, on minimal treatment and off steroids, with no aggressive bowel flare-ups.

When I met her gastroenterologist a few years later, we discussed Brenda's case. I asked him how he felt about homeopathy. He answered, 'My feeling about homeopathy? Gratitude. Sheer gratitude.'

Jason

Jason was a twenty-two-year-old man with severe depression. He was a gentle, kind man who got on well with others, yet he had made serious attempts to take his own life on two occasions. He was on maximum anti-depressant medication. He lived on his own and worked in a local supermarket. He had no contact with his family. He had been under regular review by the excellent local psychiatric team since the age of eighteen, when he had revealed that as a child he had been repeatedly sexually abused by a family friend. The abuse began when he was six years old and continued for three years, until the man moved away. He hated it, he knew it was wrong, but his abuser had told Jason that he would kill him if he told anyone. His family had seemingly noticed nothing. He felt defenceless and terrified, and although he did everything to avoid the abuser, still the abuse happened.

Jason said that whenever the man abused him 'I would send the good part of me away out of the room, so then the abuse only happened to the bad part of me. Every time it happened I would do that. That way I kept one part of me safe.'

Although the abuse stopped when he was nine, Jason grew up severely damaged. His coping strategy for dealing with the abuse had been effective at the time, but now he continued to experience himself as being split into 'a good self' and 'a bad self'. His 'good self' could get him to work each morning and could relate fairly normally with others, but he felt his 'bad self' was so soiled, so disgusting, that he once said to me, 'If I could tear off all my skin, I would.' Once, when I asked him about his suicidal thoughts, he replied with some of the saddest words I have ever heard as a doctor: 'It's not that I want to die. It's just that I don't feel I deserve to live. There's a difference.'

I was in regular contact with Jason's psychiatrist. We both agreed that Jason was a high suicide risk, yet past psychiatric admissions had not proved helpful. Jason was one of those patients who I worried about, and with good reason. After one evening consultation I felt particularly concerned. I was not sure he could go on living with a self he so despised for very much longer. He had tried every anti-depressant and had had high-quality long-term psychiatric input. The psychiatrist agreed that the conventional therapeutic cupboard was bare. With Jason's suicide risk so high (and having recently witnessed such unexpected improvement in another patient from homeopathy) I suggested a referral to the Glasgow Homeopathic Hospital, to which Jason agreed. In response to my referral letter, the hospital asked Jason to go in as an inpatient for a few days. Jason declined. He said he was prepared to attend an outpatient appointment but saw no point in yet another futile hospital stay that changed nothing. Neither Jason's expectations, nor in truth my own, were high.

Well

Jason was seen by a homeopathic doctor at a one-hour appointment and given the remedy Anacardium[1]. Initially, Jason said he wasn't sure he'd bother taking the remedy. He said he had not found the consultation in Glasgow useful, that he found it much easier to speak with me than with a strange doctor who did not know him. I suggested he just take the remedy anyway, since it would do no harm. Two weeks later Jason came in. He looked different. He had taken the three Anacardium tablets one week ago. He said that for the first time he could remember he had been able to sit in the waiting room without feeling he was contaminating other patients. There was more. The day after taking the Anacardium he said he had glanced at his body in the shower and thought (for the first time he could remember) that it looked okay. 'Okay' was a word I had never heard Jason use about himself. In fact I could hardly dare believe he was beginning to feel that way, but the healing continued. Over the next few months it was as if Jason gently reintegrated – that's the only way I can describe it: a slow coming-together of those two parts that had separated at the age of six, under such appalling circumstances, into a good part and a bad part. I didn't stop Jason's anti-depressants – he did, and only told me a month later. He simply said he knew he didn't need them any more. It was clear he didn't. Over the next year he got promoted at work, and truly began to enjoy life. I was in touch with him occasionally over the following six years. He stayed mentally and physically well, delightfully so. He was very clear in himself that all the healing began after three carefully chosen tablets of … nothing? It was clear it was time for me to change my view of homeopathy.

★ ★ ★

Homeopathy offends conventional scientific thinking. Pharmacologists say in exasperation, 'But there's no active ingredient present in the remedy! It can't work.' Until I met these two remarkable patients I, too, shared that 'scientific' view. But these were two patients with severe pathology for whom no conventional drug was working; and both of them made dramatic, unexpected and complete recoveries only after taking a carefully chosen remedy that conventional science claimed *had* to be inactive. Was it possible that conventional science's view of homeopathy was limited, and maybe should expand to allow in fresh evidence?

I felt it would have been deeply *unscientific* of me to dismiss the evidence of these two patients. Without homeopathy, it was clear to all the doctors involved (none of whom were 'believers' in homeopathy) that one patient would have required major surgery and lived with a bag on her stomach for the rest of her life, and the other patient would have carried on living in misery with continued risk of suicide.

These were not anecdotal cases. Surely the action of homeopathy in both cases merited the title of 'evidence'? It did to me. Yet modern quantitative medical research refuses to allow as evidence anything other than a sufficiently populated controlled trial (where a group of similar patients is split in half, with one half receiving a treatment and the other a placebo). Such trials are excellent for gathering evidence for a treatment for a specific *disease*. However, a treatment like homeopathy, which is based on prescribing a carefully selected remedy that matches each unique, individual case, can never be tested by such methods. With homeopathy, a group of a hundred similar patients simply does not exist.

Does that mean that Jason's and Brenda's cases are to be dismissed from any part of a body of evidence? According to current medical wisdom the answer is: 'These are only two cases. How can anything be learned from them?' I disagree. True scientific research involves observing *all* phenomena as fully and objectively as possible, dismissing none, and only then forming a working hypothesis about what is happening, then testing that hypothesis. The unexpected is the very thing we should, as scientists, pay attention to.

As the American physicist Richard Feynman said, 'The thing that doesn't fit is the thing that's the most interesting: the part that doesn't go according to what you expected.' [2] If, in 1928, Alexander Fleming had dismissed that odd clear area on a Petri dish where a bacterial colony was *not* growing, then the miracle drug Penicillin might yet be waiting to be discovered[3]. Fleming was intrigued, stopped and asked himself how something as unexpected as that could occur – bacterial cultures usually filled and clouded *all* the agar jelly in a Petri dish. He noticed that this particular dish had been contaminated by a mould fungus, and also that the only area free of bacterial growth was around the growing fungus. He did experiments and discovered that bacterial growth was *always* inhibited beside this particular fungus. And so Fleming went on to produce the first supplies of Penicillin, the antibiotic that was to save so many lives in the Second World War, and countless millions of lives thereafter. Now that's something to say 'Well!' about.

I could not dismiss the evidence of these homeopathic remedies seemingly having had such a remarkable effect in two seriously ill patients. I wanted to know more. So I looked more closely into homeopathy. I discovered that the remedies were made by vigorously shaking or 'succussing' increasing dilutions of each substance. Following the succussion process, homeopaths found these increased 'dilutions' to be more therapeutically effective in practice, and therefore refer to them as 'higher potencies'. This seemed plain Alice-in-Wonderland to me, but having witnessed both Brenda's and Jason's suffering over many years, and having closely observed their undeniable and sustained recoveries, I put my scepticism on hold and decided to attend a course at the Glasgow Homeopathic Hospital. I was impressed by the doctors I met there: they were good clinicians. I liked the way they were with their patients. They listened with great care to each person because only a remedy that exactly matches a particular patient's illness and their whole way of being will be of help to that patient. I liked that precision – it felt right. However, I didn't like discovering that there were over two thousand remedies to get to know and then to choose from. What had I got myself into?

I continued attending courses and started travelling out to Mumbai once a year for seminars with Rajan Sankaran, a well-known and highly innovative homeopathic doctor and teacher. His teaching was inspiring. I became more confident about prescribing homeopathic remedies in my own practice when conventional treatment hadn't worked. As a GP, I always felt my first task was to diagnose serious disease as early as possible, and rapidly refer onwards. Like all my partners, I had only ten-minute appointments, so if a conventional prescription would help with more minor problems, I gave that. But when no conventional treatments worked, I donned my homeopathic hat.

I wish a greater number of 'conventional' doctors would accept that, until we have the answer to all illnesses, it's good to keep an open mind about complementary therapies. I trained as a homeopath not because I believed or disbelieved homeopathy. I studied and used it for the practical reason that I had witnessed homeopathic treatments work, even in the most serious cases. From personal experience I know this broad-minded approach, embracing both conventional medicine and homeopathy, was of benefit to many patients I treated, and also to myself when faced with a serious cancer recurrence.

However, I do understand the difficulty many doctors and members of the public have in giving homeopathy any credibility. Doctors are accustomed to drugs that can be proven to work against a *disease* in a wide range of patients. The difference between penicillin and a homeopathic remedy is that penicillin works against all bacteria sensitive to its action, and will act with the same power across a whole range of patients with a similar infection. Penicillin cures *the disease*, and the person then recovers from that infection. In contrast, the homeopathic remedy acts on *the person* (not the disease per se) and, if the correctly matched remedy has been given, that person's symptoms – both physical and emotional – then improve, as occurred in Jason's and Brenda's cases. I studied homeopathy for years and had many patients who experienced remarkable responses to homeopathic remedies, but I also treated many who did not. So I am uneasy when homeopaths claim that homeopathy is always effective, and equally uneasy when doctors claim that homeopathy is never effective. I greatly regret the current prejudice in Britain against homeopathy, which limits wider, gentler, and indeed cheaper, treatment possibilities for so many.

* * *

I had learned so much from Dr Rajan Sankaran over the years. I trusted him, had seen how sound his prescribing was, and had always thought that if my cancer ever recurred I would fly out to Mumbai to see him. Yet here I was in 2010 with a 10cm-diameter mass behind my breastbone, impinging on both lungs and heart. A long flight would not be wise, especially as I had no chance of getting any travel insurance.

I emailed Rajan the day after the recurrence was diagnosed, a Wednesday, to tell him about my situation, and to ask whether he would consider giving me a Skype consultation as I could not travel. He replied immediately: '3pm your time this Saturday.'

Three days later Rajan gave me two hours of his time in a lengthy Skype consultation that covered how I was feeling, what the scan had shown, past illnesses, my childhood, my likes, my dislikes, my hopes, my fears, the things that most concerned me and what I was sensitive to. Nothing about me as a person was left out. At the end I was exhausted, and he had the remedy.

Rajan is known as a world–class homeopathic doctor, with many celebrities among his patients. I knew his fees to be high, and justifiably so. At the end of the consultation

I told Rajan how immensely grateful I was to him for so generously fitting me in within a few days, and asked him where I should send payment for the appointment. He simply smiled and said, 'Mary, this only works as friend. Just get better. That will be enough reward.'

That first Skype consultation was nearly seven years ago, when I had just been told I had a maximum life expectancy of two years. In that time Rajan has only once changed my homeopathic remedy. He chooses the remedy well and stays with that remedy unless the patient shows they are in a new state, and therefore requires a different remedy. I remain very well on his treatment and am immensely grateful for it. I am also grateful for the conventional anti-oestrogen tablets that I take. I have absolutely no doubt how deeply both treatments have helped me over this time, and so grateful that the grapefruit-sized mass of 2010 reduced to the infinitely preferable size of a pea by 2015 – all on only homeopathic and anti-oestrogen therapy.

Conventional doctors attribute my good fortune to the anti-oestrogen hormone therapy alone. I know from speaking with them that they somehow airbrush out any possible effect from the homeopathic remedy. If I insist on the efficacy of homeopathy, as I do, and emphasise my deep gratitude for Dr Sankaran's expertise, I can almost see them thinking, 'Nice woman. Glad she's well. Pity she's got this naive belief that homeopathy works', as they smile indulgently back at me.

It's frustrating that not all the evidence is allowed on the table – it is certainly far from scientific. Had I agreed to the 'heroic' surgery in 2010 and survived to be well seven years later, the medical profession would undoubtedly have attributed my longer survival time to the surgeons' skill and the anti-oestrogen therapy. Yet a homeopathic remedy is not permitted to be part of my present wellbeing. I hasten to add that my own oncologist, the delightful Dr Carolyn Bedi, has a wide-open mind to whatever is of benefit. She simply smiles and says to me (as she runs her impossibly busy clinic), 'Mary, in your case, we're way out of evidence-based territory now. Whatever you're doing, just keep on doing it.'

NHS clinicians have to be magicians of time these days, simply to see and care for all the patients referred to them. Our current medical culture understandably concentrates on health *problems*. It has little time or funding with which to investigate the anomalies, where the predicted disease progression does *not* occur. My father-in-law smoked heavily for forty years and never had a cough. Whatever was going on in that pair of lungs? The dog that didn't bark the night a racehorse was stolen from the stables may have led Sherlock Holmes to solve the mystery in Conan Doyle's story *Silver Blaze,* but the medical equivalent of that dog – the patient who doesn't get the predicted symptom or whose disease mysteriously remits – is simply dismissed from the medical puzzle and allowed to play no part in the solution.

As a young medical student, when the florid inflammatory arthritis from my teenage years finally eased off, I was simply discharged. Yet only four years previously the senior rheumatologist treating my second acute flare-up had written to my GP saying, 'I am afraid the prognosis for this young woman is very poor indeed.' I knew I had their good will, but I couldn't understand why the rheumatology doctors at the Northern General didn't want to know what might have led to my symptoms settling. Our culture is still so *disease*-orientated that when a patient gets unexpectedly better they are labelled as having a 'spontaneous remission' (whatever that is) and rapidly discharged from the clinic – one less mouth to feed drugs into. They simply drop off the medical radar.

When Alexander Fleming saw that anomaly in that Petri dish, his response was, 'That's funny', and he investigated – with invaluable results. Today we medics never seem to have time to follow through on the question, 'Now how did that happen? Why did that patient get better?' Isn't it funny that we don't?

In just the same way now, with a cancer that I was expected to die from five years ago, no research team is contacting me to see whether anything I am doing is contributing to my good health, whether anything useful can be learnt from my story that might benefit another patient. The medical radio is silent. No enquiries are made.

I sometimes wonder whether we doctors would discover that penicillin in the Petri dish if it happened now.

Eight

Ways of Living with Dying

Advances in medical technology now allow us to hope in situations where before we could only fear. A colleague who specialises in intensive care tells me of treatment advances beyond my wildest dreams as a junior doctor forty years ago. She tells me of patients going home with excellent function ten days after massive surgery because their operative and post-operative care has been so good at every stage: early organ failure is spotted immediately, infusions stimulate failing hearts, ventilators relieve failing lungs, renal dialysis rests struggling kidneys, ECMO machines allow the heart and lungs to rest (by pumping and oxygenating the blood outside the body), and filters remove toxins that would otherwise overwhelm the system. My friend tells me of her joy in being part of the team that enables so many patients to make remarkable recoveries.

She also tells me of frail elderly patients who are admitted with severe brain injuries, often from something as simple as a fall while on anti-coagulant medication; of young people in road traffic accidents who are admitted with horrendous injuries; of people with serious depression who have nearly succeeded in taking their own lives yet who still have a heartbeat on admission. Barely functioning bodies are now supported with such technical expertise that many such patients now survive. Wonderfully, some who would surely have died when I was a young doctor go on to make good recoveries. Some inevitably die, just as they did in my day. Some tragically do not recover but continue to live on, in a body and brain that barely functions.

This is where we are in the twenty-first century. Much to celebrate, much to perplex, much still to grieve. It is simply how living and dying are at this moment in the Western world. As medicine discovers more about the body, average life expectancy rises. With each welcome medical advance another procedure or treatment becomes available. As treatment possibilities soar, so do patients' expectations. As the panoply of interventions increases, doctors intervene more. How can we not? As doctors we enthusiastically share with patients not only the belief, but also the experience, that this is indeed a time of 'medical wonders'. Thirty years ago many patients died of cardiac arrest or experienced crippling heart failure after suffering a heart attack. Nowadays a stent (a small tube) is swiftly introduced into the blocked coronary artery to keep it open. The myocardial infarction (the death of a portion of heart muscle due to blocked off blood supply) is in effect aborted. Such patients often go home well the next day, blissfully unaware of the miserable fate their predecessors suffered only a few decades earlier.

Optimism grows that medical answers are there for all eventualities. Patients come to expect that doctors will be able to put all problems right. Doctors wish that they could. When our overwhelming wish to avoid illness and dying meets medical advances fuelled by political hype, hopeful expectations turn into a sense of entitlement, a feeling that 'Medicine *must* have an answer for my problem.' This varies in degree from country to country. Ian Morrison, a consultant specialising in future healthcare, grew up in Scotland, worked in Canada and now lives in California.

He comments, 'The Scots see death as imminent. Canadians see death as inevitable. And Californians see death as optional.'

Such assumptions, that death can always be delayed, only complicate our suffering when the point in an illness is reached where there are no further medical solutions. Suddenly both patients and doctors can find themselves in a minefield of failed expectations. Patients can feel angry, alone and let down, and may fear that their medical team is lacking in the necessary expertise. It is always a difficult moment when the medical team has to say that the therapeutic cupboard is bare; that further intervention is unlikely to help, and might even harm. When doctors do gently share such facts, many patients understand and accept, but sometimes the patient or the family respond angrily to such unwelcome news and insist that aggressive treatment must be continued, implying that withdrawal of treatment would be wrong.

At other times the patient may feel enough is enough, having themselves reached a place of deep acceptance, but when he or she sees that the rest of their family has not yet arrived at that place, the patient may continue with aggressive treatment either for their family's sake or simply because they themselves are too tired to have an argument about it. Some patients even continue treatment because they feel it would be letting down their medical team to 'give up' and cease fighting. Sometimes it is the family who see and accept the wider picture and it's the patient who won't give up, who wishes to persist with treatment however slim the odds of it helping. In the case of a cancer patient this can mean they continue on a regime that seriously lessens the quality of their remaining days. As a family doctor I have seen all these scenarios in palliative care. I have also witnessed the great strides made by the hospice movement in helping us all to come to terms with terminal illness in ourselves or in our loved ones.

Looking death in the eye

We all want to be happy and avoid suffering. We also know that we are content and happy when we are in an environment where we feel safe and at ease, where there are no overt threats. All of us are edgy and unhappy when we find ourselves in an environment that is fearful and threatening, and we are deeply unhappy when we have to meet the ultimate threat – our own death or that of a loved one.

Human beings respond to threatening situations in myriad creative ways. We can deny that the threat is there at all, making it possible to do nothing and stay put, with our eyes tightly shut and our fingers firmly in our ears (*freeze and hide*); we can acknowledge that the threat is real and either fight it or up sticks and move away from it (*fight or flight*); or we can resign ourselves to the fact that the threat is there, realise it is inescapable but at the same time create numerous exciting distractions, compelling and competing life scenarios that mean we don't have to dwell on the fearful situation (instead focussing our attention on pleasurable things, people and situations).

All of the above responses, and mixtures of them, are valid responses to threat. They serve us adequately at times when the threat can be ignored, moved away from, battled with or forgotten about in a plethora of other activities. They serve us less well when the threat of death is imminent either for ourselves or for those we love. And whatever tactic we have become accustomed to using when meeting or avoiding difficult situations throughout our life, this is likely to be the one waiting for us at the time of death. Because this is the one we have practised.

We are creatures of habit. As Kurt Vonnegut said, 'We are what we pretend to be so we must be careful about what we pretend to be.' [1] If our habit is to deny the difficult in life, we deny it in death also. If our habit is to turn and run from problems, then we will mentally check out when bad news comes. If distraction is our modus vivendi then we set up every alternative scenario under the sun when told difficult news. How do I know this? Because I myself have used variations of all these methods myself. It is natural to do so. It is also natural to find that in the face of imminent death none of them work, or only work for so long, and only through the expenditure of an inordinate amount of energy. You reach a point where, either through grace or weariness, you become so exhausted that you simply drop all ploys. That's when acceptance can slip in unnoticed. We are creatures of habit, but we are also creatures who can change our habits.

Capsize – the moment of surrender

One of my friends is a keen sailor. She describes the joy and excitement of racing her Enterprise dinghy around a set course – the thrill of perfectly positioning her boat to pass tightly round the mark while screaming 'Water!' at any rival's poorly placed boat, which must then give way. She describes how she overtakes competitors by keeping the maximum amount of sail up to gather the wind's force while countering the ever-increasing tilt of her boat, she and her crew leaning further and further out on the other side. She gives such a vivid picture of all the effort and rapid adjusting going on, the noise of the wind, the strain of the sails, the swell of the sea, the smack of the keel cutting through the waves, the intense, conflicting desires within her both to win the race and avoid falling into the icy Scottish waters.

Then she describes the ghastly moment when all her best laid plans fail, when maybe an extra-strong gust of wind fills the sails and she cannot let them out fast enough, when despite her now frantic efforts the slow, inexorable tipping of mast to water continues – and she capsizes. She describes the split second before the boat goes over, when everything in her is struggling ever more desperately to keep the boat upright and racing. And she describes the next moment: the quick shock of water entering wetsuit, the urgent check that both she and her crew are fine and not trapped under sail or hull, and then the sudden, surprised awareness of how peaceful it is to be bobbing in the water, all striving and racing gone, all noise of wind vanished now that the boat is still, simply floating and moving with the swell. She finds herself noticing with amazement how enjoyable this is.

As my sailing friend told me about her experience of capsizing, of the sudden peace that comes after so much struggling, I immediately recognised the moment when I had given up all my many, many ways of pushing away my full awareness of having incurable cancer. In 2010 my head knew I had incurable cancer but my heart took a while to fully accept that. A deep part of me went on rebelling and arguing with the situation. The struggle to rearrange the unrearrangeable into something more palatable was intense and ongoing. Yet suddenly the moment came when, quite simply, I capsized. The force of the facts overwhelmed my striving, all pretence at control was ripped from my hands, and I gave in.

I had been avoiding this moment so desperately only because I thought to let go would be unbearable. Yet paradoxically, just as with my friend's experience of capsize, I found it was not as bad as I had feared. Nothing dreadful happened; instead, relaxation eased in. It was so much more peaceful than what had gone before. It is almost impossible to communicate to others the surprise and the relief of this moment of surrender. They can mistakenly interpret it as bravery in an ongoing battle when in fact it is the very opposite. Courage is involved, but it is the courage to let go, not the courage to hang on.

One patient I cared for had a similar moment of 'capsize' followed by great peace and composure. At seventy-five, she had been diagnosed with inoperable bowel cancer which had already spread to the liver. It moved very fast. She went from good health to terminal illness within a matter of months. We were caring for her at home and were gradually increasing her daily morphine dose as her stomach discomfort increased.

She was a quiet woman who had received the diagnosis stoi-
cally and had not wished to go into too much discussion
about the future, about pain relief or about how long she
might or might not have to live.

One morning I went in to find her husband very upset.
He told me with embarrassment that they'd had a dreadful
weekend. She had become increasingly agitated although
not in any particular pain. Eventually when she became
almost hysterical with weeping, the duty doctor had been
called and had given her a sedating injection. I went upstairs
to her bedroom. She was sitting in bed, looking almost
sheepish. She apologised profusely for having created such
a stir. I told her she had every reason to create any amount
of stir any time she liked, given all that she'd had to adjust
to recently. I was glad she had been able to let out her full
emotions. I asked, 'How does it feel to have let all those
feelings through? It must have taken some courage.' She
looked at me in surprise and, given permission, did indeed
check how she now felt. A slow smile spread across her face
as she said, 'It feels rather good. It's such a relief. It feels as if
the cat's out of the bag at last!'

I smiled with her and asked, given that the cat was now
well and truly out of the bag, what worried her most. She
answered to my surprise that her greatest fear was not the
fear of dying. She could accept that. Her overwhelming fear
was that we would not be able to relieve her pain. Until she
had let the tsunami of her pent-up feelings through, she
had not been able to voice her worst fear to us, her carers.
I had explained at the time of diagnosis how we would
always give her enough morphine to deal with any pain,
but in her stoicism and shock she had not asked for more

detail at that time. Over the past few weeks, as her pain had increased and the daily dose of morphine rose, she had become intensely worried that we would run out of pain relief and would not be able to relieve more severe pain as the cancer progressed.

Thanks to her new openness I was able to tell her with great confidence that our team was superb at pain relief. I remember using the term 'We're second to none' and meaning it, so good were our nurses. I told her that morphine was such a wonderful pain-reliever. I described how her current dose would gradually be increased over the coming weeks as her body acclimatised to it. I assured her that we would not follow behind her pain but would always up the twice-daily slow-release morphine enough to deal with any pain she might have. I promised she would always have a supply of morphine syrup in the house that she could take herself for any unexpected pain. Her relief was palpable. Our meetings became relaxed after this, as did her relationship with her family. She died peacefully at home, all pain controlled, a few months later.

Ways of dying

Over the thirty years that I have practised as both a hospital doctor and a general practitioner I have seen many people die. As a general practitioner I've been part of a team of doctors and excellent district nurses giving palliative home care to patients with cancer. It was a privilege to care for these patients. While there is no right or wrong way to die, I saw that some ways of meeting death involve less suffering while some ways involve more.

I found that the majority of patients moved towards a deeper acceptance of their situation and I can honestly say that these patients, and their families, suffered less.

Once the fear of death had been acknowledged, life seemed paradoxically to become easier. However, those patients with terminal cancer who had great difficulty accepting their diagnosis tended to suffer more. They could not talk freely with their families or with us about what mattered to them so their anxiety levels tended to remain high and their treatment choices sometimes generated greater stress. The two groups showed equal bravery, and there is no right or wrong way to be. Simply, one group seemed to suffer less.

It is so very hard to get it right as carers, too. Sensitivity to the patient's wishes has to be the guide. Yet we need to be gentle with ourselves and with each other (whether we are a family member, friend, doctor or nurse) as we err either on the side of too much bluntness about the situation, or too little. Some patients quietly accept their situation at a deeper level of awareness than that of their medical staff. They live, and continue to wish to live, without any need for deep discussions with medical carers. Each person is different and the only guideline is to follow the lead of the patient.

Dark days
In telling my story I have emphasised the relief that comes in allowing everything to be just as it is. It's tempting to then write only about the joy of the good days, but that would not be the full picture. The good days are only so good, so free, because the bad days are allowed to be just as they are too, without any manipulation or suppression.

Here is a diary entry from one of my difficult days.

August 2015

I woke this morning with the aching in my breastbone again. It's not a severe pain. It never physically stops me doing anything. I know to be grateful to still be alive and well five years after cancer recurrence was diagnosed. But when you know from every scan that cancer is definitely present in a part of your body, and that part then gives you pain, even a dull ache can be commanding. My mind goes back to an extraordinary exhibition I saw several years ago at the Baltic Centre in Newcastle. It consisted of assembled human bones dug up from a long-ago war grave. I remember wondering about the ethics of it at the time. It was shockingly poignant to see so many carefully collected, no-longer-needed bones exhibited together in rows of like type: thighbones, neckbones, armbones, breastbones. The variation in length, strength and thickness of adjacent bones told its own tale, yet all the diverse beings whose bones these were had died and been buried in the same tumbled grave.

My own cancer recurrence was just then newly diagnosed, my only symptom an intermittent sternal ache. Having just declined a replacement sternum I couldn't help but wonder how long my own diseased breastbone would continue to hold my ribs together. My mind would roam into anxious future scenarios about how death might come. Would I spring open like the ribs of an old boat that fall away from their beached keel?

Having a sharpened awareness of both mortality and bone structure, I felt an odd affinity with the long-dead

111

owners of these assorted skeletons. I wanted all these human bones to be laid respectfully back in their grave, not exposed as an art form to the gaze of casual eyes. My own eye was inevitably drawn to the row of breastbones. Who were the folk who had carried these over their hearts? How had they died? Some breastbones were as thin and delicate as a lobster shell while others appeared armour plated and thick. What thickness my own sternum? I hoped for the latter while sensing the former. I moved on.

Five years later the sternal ache still comes and goes. Scans over the years have not shown deterioration, but each time I experience a few days of this oddly gnawing central chest pain I wonder what is happening within my breastbone, and behind it. Surely something? I remind myself once again of Lama Yeshe's words on my visit to him five years ago, just after the cancer had recurred . . .

Entering full of fear, leaving full of laughter

I went to see Lama Yeshe soon after the recurrence was diagnosed in 2010. I felt death was probably close and, if anything, I was going to ask him for instructions about staying as calm as possible around the time of death itself. I was feeling anything but calm as I drove down the valley that morning. I was still coming to terms with the knowledge that I had such a massive tumour behind my sternum, so close to heart, lungs and other vital organs. Being a doctor definitely did not help. I could picture all the organs. While on one level I was calm, accepting and steadily trying to adjust to the fact that these might be my last few months, the truth of what I was actually feeling came straight out when I spoke to him:

'Lama Yeshe, I feel as if I have a hand grenade inside my chest. It cannot be safely removed and I don't know when it's going to go off. It's terrifying. I'm not even sure that I'm safe to be driving.'

To my surprise, he responded to this dramatic opener with a matter-of-fact description of his own state of health. 'When we escaped from Tibet to India, we met tuberculosis for the first time. I had a large part of one lung removed, but recovered. Then I came to Scotland and did nothing but eat your sweet diet for many years.' He chuckled as he went on to say, 'It is my karma. I earned my diabetes and now I have high blood pressure too.' Gesturing to our two, definitely no-longer perfect, bodies, he burst out laughing – his shoulders shook with it – and said, ' *Very* bad time now to identify with body: body falling apart!'

As a friend said later, 'Well *that* was saying it like it was.'

And that was the magic of it. I had shared my worst fears about a body I no longer felt safe in and Lama Yeshe had agreed, not argued, used his own failing body in solidarity and said it like it was: very bad time to identify with body.

Something happened in that moment, a shift in perspective so simple but utterly liberating. Without knowing it, I had been totally identifying with my body. In the moment he challenged that assumption, it disappeared. I had no idea *what* I fully was, but I knew instantly that I was not just this physical body. Whoever bursts out laughing on hearing his advice (and I sense many readers will have done just that) cannot be taking themselves to be only a body either, or they really wouldn't see the joke.

I had gone in to see Lama Yeshe quaking with fear and come out shaking with laughter. And that sense of acceptance and allowance has continued. Nothing about my physical condition or longevity had altered, but everything was changed. He didn't tell me to say long prayers or mantras. He didn't ask me to join up. He didn't give me instructions for the time of dying. He didn't suggest I might live longer than I was assuming. He simply pointed out that now of all times was not a good time to identify with the body. Only then did I realise how intensely I had been doing just that. Only then did I realise how much suffering such tight identification with the physical body brings with it. Somehow when you speak with Lama Yeshe there is much more spaciousness, much more room for *not knowing* what we truly are, much more generosity of vision. In a larger space, problems appear smaller. And because Lama Yeshe *is* that spaciousness, you cannot help but share it. I had not realised how contracted my view of myself had become – a view which focussed on *my* body, *my* illness, *my* death – until he blew it open.

My spontaneous reaction to his wisdom was to join in with the laughter and let go. He didn't make me do that, nor did I try to do that. It simply happened. He himself is fearless, so you cannot help but catch some of the same. The sense of freedom and gratitude is then overwhelming.

A wise Malawian woman suffering from HIV/AIDS told her doctor, 'When you get AIDS there are two illnesses. The first illness is the problems and pains that you suffer with HIV. You have to deal with that. The second illness is the fear of what HIV will do to you in the future. It is very important not to catch the second illness.'

I would say that most cancer sufferers, myself included, catch the second illness. I am so grateful to Lama Yeshe for curing me not of the first illness (cancer) but of the second one – paralysing, consuming fear of what the cancer will do in the future. I do not know how he transmitted carefreeness about that to me. I am simply grateful that he did. Whenever I thank him he replies, 'You are very lucky. You do not have too much glue. I say the same to many people and it does not go in.'

As the years go by I realise that I do have 'glue', that I do have a habitual way of sticking back together my old wishful ideas, despite the evidence. An assumption that 'now I am well I will stay well' slips back in whenever I have a good spell of health. As a result I am always freshly disappointed when the sternal pain recurs and reminds me that the cancer is still actively with me ...*Does it have to be? These are the days of medical wonders, after all* . . . That is when I bring Lama Yeshe strongly to mind, remember his advice and let his words sink in deeply again. If I have a practice, this is it: to allow all the feelings, including any renewed alarm, all my keening and yearning for the cancer to go away, all my sudden anxiety for the family without me, to just *be*, and be fully felt in the context of spaciousness, immenseness and kindness that Lama Yeshe communicates and is.

I can write only of where spaciousness, acceptance and warmth opened up for me, personally, when meeting acute fear. Everyone is different and each will have his or her own unique way. For many, being in nature, being with animals, opens up the wider perspective. For some it is listening to music or reading poetry. Others access that space through cycling or running. My father would always go walking, preferably climbing the nearest high hill, in order to accept the difficult. He described his poems as 'doggerel, sheer doggerel' but we found them wonderful. In one he describes his love of climbing as 'the cult of the rising foot' and finishes with these lines:

> And I wonder how many discover
> That the mind's horizon too,
> Whatever the mood or the moment,
> Lifts with the widening view. [2]

AJ Gunn

Another entry from my diary:

April 2016

Things have changed, and changed suddenly. After nearly a full year of feeling physically well, having only occasional, very mild twinges of rib pain, suddenly last week came a deeper, sterner pain. It grew and radiated from my breastbone to my ribs. It wasn't worse on breathing in. It was worse all the time. The pain grew despite paracetamol and continued over twenty-four hours despite added codeine. It felt akin to a growing labour pain. I could remember when in labour with my second child, I felt the growing contractions and confidently thought, 'Oh yes, I know this. I can deal with this, I can breathe through this.' The same was true for this pain. It was quite bearable and breathable until, just as happened with my labour pains of long ago, suddenly it came in with boots on. Last week, when the pain suddenly became severe, I reached with gratitude for the oxycodone tablets my GP had given me the year before 'just in case'. For the first time, I needed them. I fell asleep with immense gratitude as the oxycodone dissolved the pain.

A bone scan the previous year had shown that the cancer was present in my breastbone but was unchanged from previous scans. It seemed stable. Since I then had no bone pain the oncologist had agreed with my plan to stay off tamoxifen – my last remaining anti-oestrogen option – unless, and until, persistent bone pain or other symptoms occurred. Knowing that each anti-oestrogen drug remains effective against the cancer only for a limited period (usually around two years), knowing that the effectiveness of one anti-oestrogen (arimidex) had already been 'used up', made me want to reserve taking tamoxifen only for when I really needed to. I had already taken it for eighteen months and wished to eke out any continuing effectiveness for as long a period as possible. My decision to hold off was made easier by the exhaustion and lowered mood I always experienced on the drug.

I had no doubt last week that it was time to start tamoxifen again. To my relief the deep sternal pain eased off completely on the fourth day of taking it. It seems the tamoxifen is still active against this tumour, and for that I am immensely grateful. But it is a double-edged message. The pain easing on tamoxifen tends to confirm that it was cancer in the bone, in my sternum, starting to grow again, that had caused such intense localised pain. Remaining well for so long off treatment, having come to what felt like a healthy accommodation with the cancer just being there, I had slipped into hoping that maybe the cancer cells had come into a more healthy accommodation with themselves too. A quiet optimism had grown that maybe they would not grow again for a while yet. This week I have had to accept that that is probably not the case.

Ironically, only two weeks ago I emailed my oncologist saying how well I was keeping, requesting another routine CT scan since it was now ten months since my last one. Maybe at some level I sensed trouble might be brewing again. I phoned last week and was relieved to be given an early scan date. I also emailed Dr Sankaran to arrange another Skype call (after which he gave me a new remedy).

I have now been pain-free for a week, am deeply grateful for the tamoxifen, but am already feeling the usual exhaustion and unwellness that comes from being back on the drug. It takes some of the bounce out of my gratitude to feel this unwell taking the remedy for the bone pain. Gratitude still wins out, but the flatter mood that always comes with tamoxifen flattens the gratitude as well.

When the pain came last week it felt unarguable that the cancer must be active again. I'm deeply sad to recognise and accept that. It would be so good if it just continued staying dormant. Could the cancer cells not just forget their fall into chaotic growth, could they not just be welcomed back into healthy cell behaviour? I would so love it if they could. Besides, I'm being such a 'good', accepting patient. Could illness not just pass me by, just quietly not notice me? Could it not just skip me, just this once? I truly have had such a lovely time in the wings, offstage, not being ill and being off all treatment, that I find myself very reluctant to be called back onstage again. Sadness and foot-dragging is the overwhelming feeling, *coupled with a wry acknowledgement of how lucky I have been to date, and how much more luck I would still like, thank you very much. After a day's glorious relief that the intense pain had vanished, I'm left feeling a bit vacant and nonplussed while waiting for the scan. I don't feel anxious or tense. I simply feel tired, deeply tired.*

When the pain was severe last week I found I could say the straightforward Buddhist prayer that covers all eventualities, and say it from my heart:

If it is better for me to be ill, may I be ill.
If it is better for me to be healed, may I be healed.
If it is better for me to die, may I die.

All is accepted, while no outcome is ruled out. When the pain was strong I could say the second and third lines wholeheartedly, albeit with a strong preference for the second line. To my surprise it was the first line I felt the most resistance to. I found I could say, 'If it is better for me to be ill, may I be ill' but had to immediately qualify it with a fervent 'but not ill for too long. It's so dreary and tiring for all concerned, most especially for the ill one.'

Allowing all feelings to be, I realise I'm more than sad. Although it would be lovely if the CT scan next week shows no growth, I doubt that it will.[3] A line from a guided meditation comes back vividly. At a retreat in Portugal last summer (with the Advaita Vedanta guru Mooji), I was quietly dozing off during one guided meditation. I suddenly came to when Mooji said, 'And if you feel self pity at this point, you will plummet.' Although I missed the context, that line woke me up and felt relevant. I sensed the difference between feeling tender, kindly compassion towards myself and feeling pity. Pity has a sharpness to it. If I feel pity towards myself I must somehow see myself as pitiable.

A part of me responds defiantly with, 'Well, why not? Who wouldn't feel sorry for themselves if they suddenly discover that their cancer is regrowing and the treatment cupboard is nearly bare? Why should I deny this feeling of self-pity? Get real; it's okay to feel sorry for yourself at such a time. I'm done with being brave and acting as if it's all alright. It's not.'

I watched the argument between 'self-pity dangerous' and 'WTF – self-pity unavoidable' play out in me for a while. Then I noticed that in the watching was tenderness, burgeoning tenderness. A tenderness that saw how hard it is for me or anyone else to be in such a sticky position, and a tenderness that also saw the wisdom in being aware of, and also wary of, letting self-pity take centre stage at such a moment. Instead, the watching tenderness grew and took centre place.

Uninterfered with, it became boundless. A warmth of feeling that included everything and couldn't be limited. And I wasn't doing it.

On writing that last line, giving birth to my children comes to mind for a second time. I remember that when the midwives told me to push, I pushed with the best of them. I turned red in the face, holding my breath, giving my idea of pushing everything I had. I wanted this baby born; I had been in labour many hours. The midwives warmly encouraged my strenuous efforts. To my surprise, despite pushing mightily with each contraction, very little happened. My baby's head simply did not move down . . . I began to hear the clank of obstetric forceps in the background. Then, more from sheer exhaustion than from planning, came a contraction when I relaxed, and in that moment I felt my baby's head moving downwards through the birth canal. With ease and purpose. And I wasn't doing it. It was an allowing rather than a forcing of anything. It was a movement free of effort. In that moment I discovered that my body knew how to let be and let go of this baby – my head just needed to keep out of it. My idea of pushing had been hindering a natural-ness that was ready and waiting to birth this baby. Relieved cheers from anxious midwives erupted as the head crowned, and my beautiful baby was born after only another few contractions experienced in this way.

That phrase 'And I wasn't doing it' is the simplest way I can find of describing such moments – precious moments when something entirely natural in us, an energy we maybe have not consciously known before (but on becoming aware of, instantly know to be trustworthy) takes over. We are so often taken up with 'doing' that we forget to allow any room for simply 'being'. Although I am not readily sensi-tive to music, I occasionally go to concerts. When I look at the rapt expression on the faces of some concert-goers, in that moment I sense that they are experiencing something similar. Each one of us finds our own opening. For my dad (tone deaf with zero sensitivity to music) it occurred when climbing his beloved mountains. It is difficult to capture in words, but Dad slipped the sense of it into his poems, as in

Well

this one, written after a glorious lone mountain climb in the Highlands one spring day:

> Blue sky, aspiring to the blue of ocean,
> High-rearing mountains mirrored in the bay,
> Sea, wood and hill are here in rare conjunction,
> For this is Torridon, and this is May.
>
> The river far below has fallen soundless,
> A sense of utter stillness fills the air,
> While all around extends serene and boundless
> A beauty richer than the eye can bear.
>
> And how can words that halt and lines that stumble
> Recall the splendour of a treasured day?
> Then let it pass – be thankful and be humble
> To walk the hills of Torridon, in May.
>
> Magic of desert dawn, of Arctic twilight,
> Of wilder summits half the world away,
> But I remember mountains nearer, dearer,
> I will remember Torridon, in May. [4]

AJ Gunn

Nine

Dying Into Living

'All my life I have felt like a caterpillar.'

Well *that* got the congregation's attention. Neat, impeccably dressed Father MacLean giving his weekly homily from the pulpit – a caterpillar? Adam and Rebecca stopped shuffling in the pew beside me. Suddenly Sunday mass had got interesting.

'Caterpillars cannot do very much. They move by hunching themselves up. They spend their lives moving slowly across leaves, eating them,' Father MacLean continued, 'But you can't tell me that somewhere, deep inside every caterpillar, there isn't a sense of some greater possibility. Although they cannot know what it is to be a butterfly (until they become one), in their life as a caterpillar they must somewhere hold a sense of delight at an amazing potential within them, a way of being that is beyond their wildest dreams. Well, that is how I feel about life on this earth. Life here can often be clumsy and difficult, a struggle to get through each day. But I know that deep within each one of us is an amazing possibility. Although I feel like a caterpillar in my life here on earth, I know that I also have a different, unimaginably greater possibility within me. I know that when I die I will meet Our Lord in heaven, and there happiness is complete.'

Stretching this analogy, one could say that the Christian church has traditionally taught that we are all caterpillars (in the case of some schools of Christianity pretty miserable and undeserving caterpillars at that) who nonetheless can be redeemed and transformed into beautiful butterflies. In contrast, the Buddha taught the same story from the other end. He taught that we are all perfect butterflies already, every single one of us. No redemption required. Our only problem is that we are butterflies who have completely forgotten what we are, and instead keep insisting that we are caterpillars, and so continue to act in very limited ways.

The Jesuit teacher Anthony de Mello (1931–1987) was the director of the Sadhana Institute, a centre of spiritual learning, in Poona, India. He was known for his inspirational teaching, which incorporated both Christian and Buddhist perspectives. He would sometimes begin his seminars by telling the following story. Once, an eagle's egg was placed by mistake in the nest of a farmyard hen. The baby eagle hatched and grew up with the hen's chicks. All his life he behaved like them, pecking the ground for food and every now and then fluttering his wings ineffectually like they did but never taking off into the air. Then, one day, he looked up and saw a wonderful golden bird flying high above the farmyard. The eagle-chick asked the hen-chicks around him, 'What is that bird?'

'"That's the eagle, the king of the birds," said his neighbours. "He belongs to the sky. We belong to the earth

– we're chickens." So the eagle lived and died a chicken, for that's what he thought he was.'[1]

Tony de Mello would then look straight at his audience and tell them that this story was about them; that they too were eagles pretending to be hens. His message was that in truth we are all golden eagles unaware of the heights to which we can soar. His book *Awareness* is all about waking up to that fact. It is about meeting and befriending the anger and fright that keeps us imprisoned within our painfully limited view of ourselves, our painfully limited view of the world. He describes each one of us as being 'the prisoner, the prison and the prison-guard.' It's an inside game. We do it to ourselves. But if we *do* it, then the good news is that we can *un-do* it. How to change? How to grow into who we really are? The second part of this book offers ways of doing that, ways of letting our 'old self' die, so that who we really are can begin to live and move and have its being.

All we need do is to open the door on our fixed ways of seeing and behaving, look at them and see if these ways truly serve us best. If they are not serving our happiness, if we see that in fact they are limiting us, then we are free to allow wider, kinder ways of being to develop and take their place. All we need do is to start opening the inner doors that we took to be walls.

The Door
Go and open the door.
   Maybe outside there's
   a tree, or a wood,
   a garden,
   or a magic city.

Well

Go and open the door.
    Maybe a dog's rummaging.
    Maybe you'll see a face,
or an eye
or the picture
    of a picture.

Go and open the door.
    If there's a fog
    it will clear.

Go and open the door.
    Even if there's only
    the darkness ticking,
    even if there's only
    the hollow wind,
    even if
        nothing
          is there,
go and open the door.

At least
there'll be
a draught. [2]

Miroslav Holub (1923–1998)
Reproduced with kind permission
from Bloodaxe Books.

Part Two

Changing
Perspectives

So what is it that stops us from opening the doors, looking at a different view, and feeling the draught? Fear. Part One tells my personal story about encountering fear. Part Two describes the help I was given to meet that fear. When I put this help into practice I found that my fear dramatically reduced. Fear is personal, but the help available for meeting fear is universal. At heart, all the different methods ask us first to look at how we view our life, as this determines how we then respond to life's events. When our view shifts, everything changes. If our view tightens, everything becomes more difficult. If our view opens, everything relaxes. Life continues to be just as eventful but our journey through it becomes easier. Part Two describes the tools for first discovering what our routine view is and then gently allowing it to become more closely aligned with what is – with the actual circumstances in our life and in the world. We find that we live more freely and vividly when we are no longer in conflict with what is.

One

How Do We Look At Our Life?

How we perceive the world around us determines the sort of life we lead. And the way we perceive the world is in itself determined by our experiences in life, especially our experiences when young. If we have been brought up in a loving environment, given a safe space as children to discover our own abilities to meet difficulties, then as adults we are more likely to have a fairly happy and confident take on life. We will lead a very different life to that of a person who was brought up in a fearful environment by anxious parents who were perhaps unable to give their child any sense of his or her own capacity to meet and survive difficulties. As an adult, that second person may well have a timid and fearful take on life. Or, if we have been brought up in an angry and aggressive environment where only success counts, we may as adults bulldoze those around us in our ingrained need always to be the winner. On the other hand, if our parents brought us up to be unfailingly peaceful, to always avoid confrontation, then we may as adults lead a rather downtrodden life. It is worth examining our own routine 'take' on life because it largely creates the world we inhabit.

The way we feel and think always comes through in the way we act and speak. The way we feel and think also has a habit of confirming itself, perpetuating itself. If we perceive the world as always too small, we will feel continuously confined in it, and our view of smallness is confirmed. If we have a fixed view of the world as full of potential persecutors, then our role is that of victim, and we will spend our lives fighting, appeasing or escaping our perceived persecutors. If we see the world as a scary, combative arena where we must always be strong or we're done for, then we're likely to wear armour and have verbal missiles ready to throw. When these missiles land, others may be quick to confirm our view that the world is indeed an aggressive place, requiring us to up the retaliation, and our life becomes an arms race. If, on the other hand, we have a fixed Pollyanna-type view that the world is always nice and everyone means well, we will insist on all our experiences in life being amicable, and may gloss over threatening behaviour that we would be wise to defend ourselves against. The problem lies not so much in our specific take, or perspective, but in the *fixity* of that take.

If our inner motivation is self-righteous anger then, even if we act in the cause of world peace, the seeds we sow in the world will be angry ones. If we are moved only by kindness and compassion, we will plant very different seeds in our self and in others. We all broadcast our inner state, and leave its long wake behind us in the world.

Our perspective on the world can remain both unexamined and unchanged for a long time. Yet circumstances are always changing around us. Charles Darwin's studies in evolution confirmed that those species which best adjust and adapt to changing environments are the species that best survive and thrive.

All of us tend to carry a hidden fixity of view of which we ourselves may be quite unaware. It takes a challenge, a shock, to waken us to our own fixity. The eighteenth-century philosopher Immanuel Kant said that it was only reading the writings of his contemporary David Hume that awoke his mind from its 'dogmatic slumber'. [1] For me, a sudden diagnosis of cancer let me know just how dogmatically I myself had been slumbering. Suddenly my world, with all its expectations and sleepy dogmas was, quite literally, rudely awoken. Our fixity of view is only so powerful, so difficult to loosen, because we are barely aware of it. We are so very accustomed to it. This sleepy stuckness limits us and keeps us under the impression that our routine take is the only view possible. It often takes something quite 'rude' to shake us out of it.

How my own take on illness evolved and changed

As the behaviour of my cancer changed over time, my perspective, or 'take' – on my own illness, and on life in general – also underwent change, in the ways described below.

Take One

When I was first diagnosed with breast cancer, my doctor-perspective (that illness mainly came to others, that I was the healthy medic who helped them) changed to patient-perspective. I viewed the lump in my breast as a group of my own cells gone rogue. I saw cancer as the enemy and I went into all out battle with it. I had the lump removed and took radiotherapy and chemotherapy to get rid of any remaining cancer cells inside me. As a mother of young children this was the right perspective for me then. With the passage of time I began to believe that the aggressive treatment had worked, that no cancer cells remained in my body.

Take Two
When I reached fifty-seven, the cancer recurred. My first take hadn't worked out; a few cancer cells had survived the aggressive treatment, in a lymph node behind my breastbone. These had grown into a 10cm-diameter mass with spread into the lung. I would have gone for surgical removal again if the benefits had outweighed the risks. They did not. My take was that I would die of this growing cancer in the next few months or years, and that I must preserve my wellness for as long as possible with gentle therapies that did not make me feel ill. I therefore took only hormone treatment and homeopathy.

Take Three
Very soon my initial calmness wore off and I started waking early, overwhelmed by the sense of having a hand grenade in my chest, right beside my heart. The suspense of not knowing when it would explode was unbearable. My unconscious take was that I *was* my body, and that my body had now become totally unreliable, indeed deeply threatening. I was living in a small, unstable, contracted world of acute fear. The suffering was intense. I went for help.

Take Four

I spoke with Lama Yeshe. In the moment that he smiled and said, 'Very bad time now to identify with body: body falling apart!' Everything – how I looked at the world, where I was looking from – shifted into a much larger space. I was no longer just little frightened me in a diseased body, being brave in a difficult world. I was still 'me in a ropey body' but I saw that I was so much more also. I didn't *think* this, I saw this, sensed this. My take or view opened into a sudden knowing that I was not just this body. If I was anything, I was the calm awareness that knew that. I saw that I didn't really know how long I would live and miraculously, in this larger much more relaxed space, that didn't seem to matter in the same way as it had. I shifted from dreading and miserably predicting the future to ... leaving it alone. The future would be as it would be. There was *this moment* to be alive in and enjoyed first. Ease, immense gratitude and a sense of ongoing possibility moved back into my life.

★ ★ ★

Each of those four 'takes' I had on my illness had their own validity, and each determined how I experienced life. Whatever our view is, that is the world that we live in. We create our own world. In Takes Three and Four my diagnosis remained exactly the same, yet there was a world of a difference between the two. Living in the world of Take Three I was the terrified victim of my own cancer. Living in the world of Take Four I was not. I was still living in a diseased body but somehow I was not defined or limited by that. I discovered with delight that a wider perspective changed everything.

Our problem is not our specific view,
  but the fixity of that view

The good news is that our fixity of view is not itself fixed, as my own story shows. What has grown up over time (our view of life, our habits) can also be shed over time. Recent research in neuroscience confirms that our brains are far more flexible and 'plastic' than scientists had previously assumed. As the neuroscientist Siegrid Löwel states, 'Neurons that fire together, wire together.' [2] Neural pathways are built up and strengthened by repetitive behaviour. We all tend to cling to certain ways of reacting, because these at least feel familiar to us, but not all habitual ways serve us well. It is our *attachment* to these habits that causes us (and our neural pathways) to remain embedded in them. The Tibetan spiritual master Tilopa said to his student Naropa over a thousand years ago, 'It is not your desire, but your clinging to desire, that is the problem. Cut through *attachment*, Naropa.' [3] Once we examine and when necessary change our habits, then seemingly fixed neural pathways fall into disuse and fade away. Only repetitive use of any pathway keeps it open.

But first we have to notice our own fixity, our own 'attachment' to a certain unexamined point of view. Personally I have found Byron Katie's method of self-inquiry to be by far the most powerful way to uncover my own fixity of view. Her 'turnarounds' are especially useful. Katie recommends that we write out on a worksheet our feelings about a difficult incident. Once we have identified one of our own strongly held fixed points of view about this incident, Katie asks us to turn our statement around to its opposite, and to switch the pronouns, and see if these turnarounds are more true, or as true, as the original statement. [4]

How Do We Look At Our Life?

For instance, on my own worksheet I wrote down my feelings about a painful incident with a friend in the past. I put, 'She should not have been so thoughtless and unkind to me.' The turnarounds to this were, 'She should have been thoughtless and unkind to me' (no, that one didn't feel true); 'I should not have been thoughtless and unkind to her' (on reflection I could see that that was *as* true – I had probably misunderstood her as deeply as she had misunderstood me); 'I should not be thoughtless and unkind to me.' *Oh, now that one rings truest of all. Here I am, months later, still ready to ruminate on my hurt feelings. In this moment just who is being 'thoughtless and unkind' to whom here? My friend is not present and our friendship has survived. Why am I rehearsing and clinging to a painful moment in the past? This is only me doing this to myself.*

By going over a past hurt in my mind (something most of us do), I saw that I was in fact firing and wiring an 'indignation pathway' which would not serve me well in the future, and without which I would be much freer. Once the futility of a habitual way of behaving is fully seen, that habit loses all power.

It's strong medicine, but it fair shakes us out of any dogmatic slumbering! It comes as a shock to realise that the opposite of a firmly held personal view might actually be truer, or that the very thing that you are angrily accusing the other of doing to you, you are in fact doing much more powerfully to yourself. Your view certainly loosens up when you see that, and so does your world.

> *The world is as you believe it to be. It can never be more or less than that.* [5]
>
> *Byron Katie*

Well

Flexible brain, flexible world
When our view of the world starts changing, so does our world.

> *We but mirror the world. All the tendencies in the outer world are to be found in the world of our body. If we could change ourselves, the tendencies in the world would also change. As a man changes his own nature, so does the attitude of the world change towards him. This is the divine mystery supreme. A wonderful thing it is and the source of our happiness. We need not wait to see what others do.* [6]
>
> *Mahatma Gandhi*

Our experience shapes how we view the world, and our view then shapes our further experiences of the world. If our view is flexible then our experience happens freely. We can be fully present and open to whatever is happening. Our life, and our view of life, remains dynamic, as life always is. When we ride the waves of life we are able to be present, flexible, relaxed and fully aligned with what is.

Two

You Cannot Step Twice
Into the Same River

Why should I change any of my habitual ways, any of my habitual views? If all is well in my own life, if all is well in the world, there is no call to change. But all is not well in the world, and all is not always well in our own individual lives. Each one of us knows that no matter how dear our loved ones or possessions may be to us, all will be left behind at the moment of death, and we have no way of knowing when that moment will be. This is not morbid. It is the simple truth. It is how things are. The world is constantly changing and we – like it or not – inevitably change with it. We can do so reluctantly, sulkily, resentfully, or we can accept that change is a given; we can embrace it and find that we then move forward through life's changes.

Living as a child in New Zealand and experiencing an earthquake, I felt the earth rising beneath me, the house shaking. I knew in my bones that even the earth itself is on the move, constantly forming and reforming. We are born, we grow old, we die. We know that these are the laws of life, yet especially in the West we have come to believe that we can override the changes of nature. We strive to delay ageing and dying indefinitely, to stop the changes of time in their tracks. We imagine we can Botox over all the cracks.

The Ancient Greeks were wiser. Two thousand five hundred years ago, the philosopher Heraclitus said, 'You cannot step twice into the same river, for other waters are ever flowing on to you.' [1] We know that a river constantly flows, is always changing. We get the metaphor and understand that the external world is always on the move, can never stay the same. Yet despite the acknowledged changefulness of everything around us, each of us somehow manages to hold on tight to an image of *ourself*, the one stepping into the changing river, as being constant. We are strangely quiet and oddly unobservant of the ongoing change that must be, that is, simultaneously occurring in our inner world, in our very self. Plutarch refers to Heraclitus, going on to say, 'It is not possible to step into the same river, or to come into contact twice with a mortal being in the same state.' [2]

SN Goenka, the Burmese-Indian teacher of Vipassana meditation (1924–2013) was very clear: 'Not only can you not step in the same river twice, the same *fellow* cannot step in the same river twice.' [3]

We are reluctant to admit to constant change in our self. It feels too undermining to allow the possibility that, from moment to moment, we are not the same person. I can feel my gut response as I write this: *Don't be ridiculous – of course I'm the same person as a moment ago.* Yet clearly, as modern photography, mirrors and our diaries all confirm, we constantly change over time. It is only logical to allow not just the river, but also the woman or man to be constantly moving, flowing, changing.

When I lived and worked in rural Africa, the shock of violent change, the frequency and rapidity of birth and death within communities, within families, within one life, within the earth itself, was undeniable. Babies were admitted with tetanus and died within hours; we could do nothing. Others, barely breathing, came into the ward with septicaemia, but with the right intravenous antibiotics made miraculous recoveries, bouncing home on their mothers' backs a week later. I would plant seeds in my garden that would grow like Jack's beanstalk almost overnight. However, if I was unable to water them the African sun baked their desiccated stalks back into the ground within days. Change there was strong, visible and unmissable. The rural African community, by necessity and culture, deeply acknowledged uncertainty and change as omnipresent in life and lived vividly and fully in the midst of it.

While Heraclitus proclaimed that all is change and that nothing abides, another Greek philosopher of that time, Parmenides, held a seemingly opposing point of view. In his poem 'The Way of Truth' Parmenides describes all that exists as being 'unborn, imperishable, whole of limb, unshaking, unendable, one and continuous.' [4] Parmenides argued that all that exists is made of what he called 'the One'; that this One is uncreated and indestructible; that it is also unchanging – all sensory evidence to the contrary being illusory. Parmenides' philosophy is relevant to date, the twentieth-century philosopher of science Karl Popper describing it as, 'the first Western deductive theory of the world ... One further step led to theoretical physics and the atomic theory.' [5]

Parmenides (for whom all was complete, unborn and

unchanging) and Heraclitus (all is relative and changing) lived in Greece in around the fifth century BC. At much the same time, the Buddha, a prince of the Shakya tribe, born in Lumbini (now Nepal), had left his palace, awoken to the nature of reality (the word *buddha* simply meaning 'awake'), and was teaching a growing group of monks that there are two truths. The Buddha described the nature of these two truths –

> **Ultimate truth** *(the underlying truth) is one and is unborn, unchanging and indestructible*
> **Relative truth** *(what we perceive with our senses) is constantly changing, impermanent, interdependent, arising and dissolving according to causes and conditions*

> *– and the Buddha taught that these two truths are one.*

It is wonderful how deep new understandings so often come through at the same time in history, in widely different cultures and continents. The history of philosophy and science is littered with instances of similarly coincidental discovery.

A changing view of 'stress'

Received medical wisdom has been that stress is bad for our health. I used to advise my patients to reduce their stress levels as much as possible. New research shows that stress is not always bad for our health. A 2012 study by University of Wisconsin researchers [6] showed that stress is bad for us only *if we think it is*. Apparently, the way we think not only governs the way we live but can also influence how long we live. 30,000 adults were asked how much stress they had experienced in the last year, and whether or not they felt that stress was bad for their health. Eight years into the study death rates of the different groups were analysed. A significantly higher death rate occurred only in the group who had experienced moderate to severe stress *and* who viewed stress as bad for their health. Surprisingly the group who had experienced moderate to severe stress but *did not view stress as bad for their health* had a lower death rate even than the non-stressed groups. It seems that stress, when met as a challenge, can even be good for our health.

Kelly McGonigal, a health psychologist at Stanford University in the US, gave an excellent TED talk on this research entitled, 'How to make stress your friend'.[7] She says she now advises her clients to think positively when they recognise the signs of stress in their body – the pounding heart, the increased respirations. She advises any of us, when stressed, to think, 'This is my body helping me rise to this challenge,' adding that, 'When you view stress in that way, your body believes you and your stress response becomes healthier.'

How we perceive a problem can significantly affect our wellbeing. This echoes my own experience of the radical difference between living the contracted view of Take Three (me as terrified victim of my cancer) and living the spaciousness of Take Four (me still in a diseased body but accepting this and not defined by it). The difference between these two takes is rather like the difference between a novice skier at the top of a black run: abject terror (*I'm going to die; get me off this steep slope – I'd rather slide down on my bottom*); and a confident skier at the top

143

of the same run: exhilaration, a sense of adventure (*This is risky and difficult. I'm not even sure I can do it, but I'm going to enjoy having a go*).

The first part of this book tells my story of living with cancer over the past twenty years. Over that time – now one third of my life – my perspective on illness and dying has evolved and changed. Using my own experience of ongoing illness as an example, it is clear that change in our habitual way of seeing is possible, often necessary, and can be enormously beneficial. As Heraclitus pointed out, we are constantly changing anyway. We live life more fully if we acknowledge that fact and live life as we are in this moment, rather than imagining ourselves still to be how we were in a past moment.

We get the same advice from the Buddhist teacher Dzogchen Ponlop Rinpoche:

> *Our entrance into this world came with a contract to leave it. So, whether you sigh with relief at the end of a torturous moment, or desperately wish some Hollywood movie-like instant could last forever, every moment comes to an end. Every story has an end, regardless of whether that end is happy or sad. Nevertheless, when a moment or a lifetime ends, we cannot argue with it. There is no room for negotiation. Recognising this reality is the way we come into contact with death in everyday life.* [8]

Many teachers emphasise the importance of dropping pretence and working with 'what is'. How else can we be truly present? One exercise Buddhist teachers recommend, for noticing both what changes in us and what does not change, is to observe an old photograph of our self from the past.

Musing on a photo from the past

It's a windy October afternoon, the gusts scattering leaves in the driveway, calling me out to sweep and clear. I delay over a pot of tea and the Sunday paper. A squall of rain strikes hard on the kitchen window. I look up to see that golden autumn sun has shifted into grey winter cloud, all in the drinking of a cup of tea. I pour another cup and grant all falling, drifting beech leaves full freedom to gloriously gather where they will. Happily deprived of gardening chores, I go in search of a lost notebook. In the corner of our lounge sits a wooden chest from Malawi. A large lamp and bowl rest serenely on its carved surface, belying the chaos within. This lovely chest has, over time, become the handy repository of our family's unthrowawayables: letters, cards, photos, diaries, notebooks and even, I discover, my dear late father-in-law's silver presentation tankards from the 1970s.

Rummaging through this Tardis-like store, I come across a clutch of photos from forty years ago, photos of myself as a young doctor in Liverpool. I look about twelve. My present sixty-four-year-old self doesn't know the people my twenty-four-year-old self is enthusiastically chatting to. Does my sixty-four-year-old self even know that twenty-four-year-old youngster, that 'me back then'? Her image is clear enough, looks right enough. She is here in my hand in black and white. I look at her bright, crease-free eyes, her bob of dark hair, her grin. She looks very familiar, and indeed is wearing a polo neck that once was mine. But who is she, this young woman in the picture? Is she 'me now', wearing a polo neck that once was mine, a body that once was mine, feeling feelings that once were mine, thinking thoughts that once were mine? Only a vague something in her smile, in her brightness, feels the same in me now. I am reminded of a delightful ninety-year-old patient who said to me while I weighed him, 'Do you know, Doctor, I am exactly the same weight I was when I was nineteen – just a completely different shape!'

As I gaze at these photos of 'me back then' – images literally from a previous century – something about my sixty-four-year-old self feels exactly the same as that youngster in the picture. I am her. Yet so much feels completely different. I am not her. I am indeed a completely different shape now, in every way. I feel no nostalgia, no desire to be her, to be twenty-four again. Rather, I feel a kindly curiosity, a tenderness, even a motherliness for this young being to whom so much is going to happen. I'm sure most of us experience similarly mixed emotions when gazing at photos of our younger self:

Surprise: *Did I ever look quite that young?*
Curiosity (for which read, memory lapse): *But whoever is that person I'm with?*
Tenderness: *I remember Dad taking that photo, and him taking ages as usual.*
Affection: *That was such a happy day.*
Aversion: *Oh dear that's me – the one smoking on the sofa with the smug expression, casually crossing her legs, in three-inch platform shoes and four-foot-wide bell-bottoms. No wonder I'm sitting down.*

Genuine puzzlement: *I remember that day. I was there at that party. Yet forty years on I am such a different person that I can hardly feel that the person in the photo is me.*

We remember our past selves, we are them, but we are also not them. Isn't that strange? To truly, directly see that we are not the self we were a year ago, a month ago, or even a minute ago. Just as the cells in our bodies replicate, grow, die and are replaced minute by minute; so too the moments in our lives come into being, are experienced vividly, then pass into memory ... but who is it who experiences all this? Who are we over time? What is it in us that does *not* change? Surely there must be some unchanging quality, some stable reference point within us, in order for us even to notice any change? Otherwise we would simply *be* the ongoing changeability without knowing.

It seems that we contain both the changeless (ie that which is not affected by time and is therefore able to note the passing of time, the happening of change) and also the ever-changing (ie that which is affected by time and is therefore always flowing and evolving). So, our lives reflect the truths of both Parmenides and Heraclitus. We are both the timeless and the time-bound. How extraordinary. No wonder we get confused. No wonder we find the paradox more than we can bear and instead plump for a fixity, a solidity which in essence we 'make believe' to be so. In a desperate desire for the world to be more straightforward, less fluid, we unconsciously project notions of being a fixed person in a definite world and live our life accordingly. We allow for changes to be happening within that world

– we have to make some compromise with reality, after all – but in general we do not fundamentally question our fixed notions regarding our own person. We often work from a perspective of the world and ourselves in it that is way past its sell-by date, that does not fit with our current circumstances.

My father wrote the following poem about the changes of time during a holiday in Audierne in Brittany, immediately after my sister's wedding. Just me and my Mum and Dad. The weather was grey and our threesome was lonesome. I was haunted by sunny memories of French family holidays from past years. I thought I was the only one missing the fun of my big sister's company but when I got back to university I received this poem from Dad with a note saying, 'I haven't sent this to Donella as she would be so moved she might just up and leave David ...'

Audierne

Autumn sunlight lacking lustre
Audierne.
Someone missing from the muster
Audierne.
Seagulls gleaming in the water,
Evening dreaming on the water,
Where I missed my elder daughter,
Audierne.

It's a place of paths diverging
Audierne.
And a case of truth emerging
Audierne.

You Cannot Step Twice Into the Same River

That we can't let life deceive us,
That we shouldn't find it grievous
That our girls grow up and leave us,
Audierne.

Now our foursome is diminished
Audierne.
And we know a chapter's finished
Audierne.
But if all the years in store
Should reflect the years before,
Then we will not ask for more
At Audierne. [9]

AJ Gunn

Many years later, on a visit to Orkney, Dad wrote another poem – this time about what persists, about what perhaps continues over time, about that odd sense of déjà vu that many of us get from time to time. Such moments come unexpectedly. Though striking, we usually dismiss them. Dad, too, dismissed his moment of déjà vu as 'pure fancy, of course'. Yet it must have been quite vivid for him to have written such a poem.

Déjà vu

When was I here before,
At Ottersgill?
The summer midnight glow
On Scapa Flow
Meets my contented eyes
And comes as no surprise;

149

Well

The tide race, rippling near,
Soothes an accustomed ear,
And there the hills of Hoy fall into place.
I know that outline, though the name rings new.

For this long lived in land
Has woven, strand by strand,
What vast and hidden web of ancestry:
A host of lives for whom
Could Time alone find room:
And memories, not our own,
Reach us from sires unknown,
The more, where mind is kin.

This sand beneath my heel
Has a familiar feel,
Remembered still though now my feet are shod.
The ancient echoes grow,
Till in my bones I know
That I was here before,
At Ottersgill. [10]

AJ Gunn

Three

What Increases Our Suffering and Lessens Our Happiness?

We all wish to be happy and avoid suffering. If we know and recognise the tendencies in ourselves that increase our suffering we can limit their development while cultivating those tendencies or habits that serve our happiness. Given that the world is always changing, what prevents us from being better aligned with the world moment by moment? What prevents our appropriate and creative response to life's ongoing changes? What limits our ease and happiness? Four things:

Fear
Fixity
Fury
Foolishness

The first obstacle to happiness: fear
– fear of living as much as fear of dying
Brother David Steindl-Rast, a marvellous spiritual teacher and Benedictine monk, describes our one basic choice in

life as being: whether to trust all that life brings and say a whole-hearted 'Yes' to life; or whether to resist and fear and instead say 'No' to much that life brings. Either way, life lives us, with or without our permission.

Brother David advises us against confusing anxiety with fear. Human anxiety, he suggests, is normal, is our natural response to seeing a narrow place ahead that we have to go through, the word anxiety coming from the Latin word *angustia* meaning tightness, narrowness. He says life is always leading us into narrow places; that, indeed, we all came into the world through a narrow place. When we look ahead and see a narrow place, it is natural to feel anxious. We can choose to say 'No' and be stopped by our anxiety; our anxiety then morphs into transfixing, catastrophising fear. Alternatively we can fully feel the anxiety but say 'Yes', responding to the difficult situation with courage and trust; we go ahead anyway. Brother David explains with delight:

> Once we courageously go through the narrow place, each narrow spot turns out to be a new birth. We cannot see that looking forward; from there we only see the narrowness ahead. But once we go through and look back, we see all the many narrow spots we have come through, and how each one was for us a new birth. [1]

My own experience is that while anxiety met and leaned into can strengthen us, shake us up, wake us up, we can also travel equally rapidly in the opposite direction – we can run away from fear and contract into ourselves. It seems only natural to try to escape something as unpleasant as fear. Our brain is wired to do just that. Jumping away is the right reaction to the oncoming car or to the dangerous snake. Our automatic 'fight or flight' reaction is perfect when the threat is something we can get away from, or that we can get away from us. But when the threat is ongoing, intimate and cannot be removed – what then? We have to somehow find a way of living with it. That's when we need help in finding a wider view, a greater spaciousness to live in, in which to hold all this.

Whatever its source, fear can only be experienced personally, individually. If our neighbour is anxious, it affects us, but we can never know quite how another's fear is for them, any more than we can experience their pain. We can simply see it on their faces and read it in their actions. But while fear is individual, the tools for dealing with fear are universal. Fear affects us all. Even if we are fortunate enough to live in a relatively safe community, the fear of old age, sickness and death can never be removed and can only be met. There are tools for calming fear, for challenging fear, for letting fear be and living with it courageously. All these are of immense value.

But to cut through to the root of fear, whatever its cause, and then to live fearlessly – only love will do. Not sentimental, clinging love. Not passionate, romantic love. Not anxious 'save the world' love. Not righteous 'fix the world' love. A much deeper, simpler love than that. A love that has no conditions or causes in order to love. A love that cannot exclude, that includes everyone. In the field of *this* love, fear loses all of its oxygen. It simply ceases. Put simply, once this unconditional love is let loose, fear doesn't stand a chance. And all the energy that once went into our helpless cycle of fearing/defending/fighting/lashing out and therefore fearing even more, is miraculously released for living.

Brother David describes such love as 'a wholehearted "yes" to life, to limitless, mutual belonging with all that is'. [2] That's a tall order. I did not know how unprepared I myself was for living together with serious threat until diagnosed with cancer. I initially said a firm 'No' to mutually belonging with this unwelcome development in my body. The fear I felt was up close and personal, as fear always is, whatever the source. The uncertainty of my situation could not be removed. Neither, as it turned out, could the cancer. Despite being a family doctor with broad experience of caring for the sick and the dying both in this country and in Africa, when it came to me – to my body, my cancer, my life, my husband, my children – I discovered I lacked the skills to live levelly. I had to seek help.

I found that help in abundance. To my amazement I discovered that it is possible to live in a climate of threat and total uncertainty without blanking it out, without blaming anyone else, without compulsively distracting myself, without pretending the problem isn't there, and without getting stuck in the fighting of it. The freedom and space that is suddenly present when fear slackens off is really rather wondrous. It is certainly unexpected.

The second obstacle to happiness: fixity

Fixity in how we perceive the world, in how we perceive others, in how we perceive ourselves. If we think we cannot change, we cannot. We only ever have as much power and flexibility *as we think we have.*

Part One of this book described my personal story. It happens to involve a disease called cancer, but in essence it is simply an account of a person journeying with fear over time and, if you like – or, as I didn't like – getting acquainted. At the start of the journey I would have described myself as an open-minded agnostic with warring streaks of scepticism and wonder about the world. That had been my fixed view for a while; a rationalist ready to be bowled over by beauty. Dramatic sunsets and horizon-stretching rainbows, preferably viewed from a mountaintop, set my heart singing. The innocent face and straight gaze of a baby, even without the miracle smile, always astonished and delighted me. Quotes from Mahatma Gandhi and Martin Luther King inspired me. Words from the Bible haunted me with their beauty. But then the sceptical scientist in me would step in, cast an angry eye over the poor, suffering world, roll up her practical sleeves and get on with trying to sort out this mess. If I did believe in a god, it was certainly one who should have arranged matters better than this. My fixed view was that this much suffering should never have been permitted in the first place. No judgments there, eh?

But then my world tilted and the suffering was in me. My attention became more focussed. I began to learn what supported and nourished me, and what didn't. Love and open-hearted acceptance did. Fear and close-minded resistance did not. But fear remained in me, intertwined with me, fixed in me. I began to realise how very little I truly knew about anything. That was a start. In Buddhism they say there are three defects students can have that prevent them from learning, growing and changing:

1.   Some students are like an upside down pot –
      the student is physically present but their mind
      is closed so that new truths cannot enter.

2. Some students are like a leaky pot – they are present, their mind is open, they can absorb teachings but are then unable to retain them.

3. Some students are like a pot containing poison – they are open, take in the teachings, but instantly combine and mix them with their own pre-existing negative views.

I seemed to tick all three boxes, or rather, pots. I was the upturned pot in that I believed my own view was good enough and didn't need much altering. I was the leaky pot in that although I was often touched by beauty and wisdom in the world, I soon moved on from them. And yes, I was the pot with poison in it, too, as any wisdom I met with I forcibly tried to merge with my pre-existing and fixed view. I had got out of the habit of looking deeply, curiously, like a child does, with fresh unclouded eyes, simply taking everything in.

> *... truth and reality begin when you no longer under-stand anything you do or know ...* [3]
>
> *Henri Matisse*

Our hidden fixity can be shaken loose by sharp sudden shocks. In difficulties we can wake up to a larger reality. We all know it. Meeting fear and deep surprise can have that effect. Suddenly the world is not as we had assumed, and we realise it may be time to reassess some of our other beliefs too. We start to unearth a whole heap of unexamined and stale assumptions that are not true and have been clouding our view of life without our noticing. It is shaky, even shocking, work, but invigorating when we follow Chögyam Trungpa's advice to 'lean into the sharp bits'.

The third obstacle to happiness: fury

A Native American story describes a young boy telling his grandmother how angry he is following a fight with a friend. His grandmother says, 'Ah yes, I know that angry feeling. You see, I have two wolves fighting in my belly. One wolf wants to make war. The other wants to make peace.' The young boy knows that wolves can sometimes fight each other to the death. He looks at his grandmother's belly in alarm: 'But grandmother,' he asks, 'Which wolf will win?' His grandmother answers, 'The one I feed.'

Which one do we feed? How do we react when life brings us unwelcome difficulties? Do we accept and find creative ways of working with what is? Or do we resist and angrily blame the world, God or ourselves (and sometimes all three) for allowing such unpleasantness to occur in our life? Do we believe our angry thoughts that tell us *This should not be happening to me*? But what sense does that argument make when this *has* happened? Why do we so readily let our hurt and fury take us to war with what *is*?

> You can argue with reality all you like for as long as you like. You'll lose, but only 100 percent of the time.
>
> *Adyashanti*

When I first heard this statement I was puzzled. Surely there are times when we shouldn't accept the status quo? It took me a while to realise that these spiritual teachers are not saying, 'Put up with an impossible situation.' Rather, they are saying, 'First accept what is, because that is what has already happened. From that full, unfurious, calm acceptance you are then free to respond in the best way possible for yourself and for everyone else involved, because you see the whole situation clearly'.

At one retreat with the Buddhist teacher Lama Rinchen, one person said to her, 'But I'm filled with righteous anger about injustice in the world. I don't want to give up my anger and I wish to act on it.'

Lama Rinchen answered, 'Yes, I agree. Your anger is justified. The question is whether we bring about the best outcome when we act on the basis of righteous anger. The conditions of the peasants at the time of the French Revolution were absolutely appalling. Their anger was entirely justified. But when the final outcome of the revolution ... was Napoleon Bonaparte ... was that really a good outcome?'

In our personal lives, when we turn away in fury from the difficulties, losses and illnesses that are an inevitable part of being human, we greatly increase our own suffering. Aversion and refusal to accept all that life brings is one of the strongest obstacles to happiness. By turning away we miss the opportunity for growth that each narrow place can bring.

I've heard patients say, 'You know, doctor, I'd much rather this illness had never come my way, but I am grateful for all it's taught me. It's opened my eyes.' I usually saw what they meant but felt they were taking rather a generous view. I thought they were putting on a brave face. However, when I became ill I found I felt exactly the same way. While wishing my own cancer a million miles away, I also wouldn't have wanted to lose the unexpected feeling of openness, aliveness, the increased appreciation of the everyday, the wider gaze. This isn't romanticising misfortune, it's just describing what happens when we drop all furious argument and let things be the way they are. There is a great relief in being fully acquainted with our own situation. Our decisions are clearer, we feel more centred, and the energy we previously expended on fight or flight is now fully available to us. Without our fury we become *more* powerful, not less. Opening up to the sorrows of life also opens us to the joys of life, and we discover we feel both more fully. In *The Book of Joy*, [4] a collection of discussions between the Dalai Lama and Archbishop Desmond Tutu, the Archbishop explains that in opening ourselves to more joy we do not avoid sorrow, but instead discover that we can 'face suffering in a way that ennobles rather than embitters. We have hardship without becoming hard. We have heartbreak without being broken.'

The fourth obstacle to happiness: foolishness

The Dalai Lama describes two types of selfishness: wise selfishness and foolish selfishness. Foolish selfishness is when we look after number one at the expense of everyone else around us. We are frightened and insecure and believe that our safety can only be secured by amassing more possessions, more power, more money, more fame, more property. But then we have to maintain all this moreness. We have to safeguard our possessions, insure our houses, maintain our bank balance, increase our power and fame. And we have to fight those who might steal these precious things from us. The task of foolish selfishness is never-ending. Our goal – of relaxed happiness and safety – is never achieved.

Wise selfishness is when we realise that we can be truly happy and at ease only when everyone around us is also happy. We see that they are just like us – that they, too, wish to be happy. We see that our happiness coexists with theirs. We see that our life and that of our neighbours are intimately interconnected. We are moved to look out for and care for others; we wish for others to be happy as well as ourselves; we acknowledge our own needs while taking into account the needs of those around us. This is wise selfishness. We have nothing to protect because we trust those around us and they trust us. Our goal – safety, ease and happiness – is achieved.

The Dalai Lama advises us to recognise and celebrate our common humanity, to recognise that we can only be truly happy when our human brothers and sisters are also happy, adding, 'This is not a spiritual thing. It is simply common sense.' He asks us to look from the perspective of our common humanity, to adopt the 'we' perspective, rather than the individual 'me' perspective. [5]

The first astronauts, and all astronauts since, report being extremely moved by seeing the Earth, this beautiful blue-and-green planet that is our home, suspended in the immensity of space. To them, from that perspective, it is clear that the Earth and all that lives and grows on earth is one interdependent whole. Biology, physics, chemistry and environmental science all confirm this truth. Once you see that view, of our planet suspended in the vastness of space, you see all life on Earth differently.

So why do we human beings still persist in somehow seeing ourselves as completely separate individuals who, at all costs, have to defend and protect ourselves from each other and a hostile world? Looking at the evolution of the human brain can help us understand this phenomenon.

Evolution of the human brain

Life on earth began in the oceans, moved out of the water and on to land, reptilian life then evolving into birds and mammals, primates, and the first human beings. Quite a journey, and one that is reflected in the structure of our complex human brain.

The oldest part of our brain, the reptilian brain, is represented by our human brain stem and cerebellum. The reptilian brain first appeared in fish roughly 500 million years ago. It enables individual survival. Our brain stem and cerebellum control life's vital functions – breathing, heart rate and balance.

The next evolution was the development of the limbic system, appearing above the brain stem in the brains of small mammals about 150 million years ago. The limbic system is the part of the brain that deals with our memories, emotions and also with stimulation and response. It takes in information directly from the eyes, ears, nose, tongue and touch organs in our skin, and collates this into our memories and habits. Our emotions and instinctual reactions arise from what we like in the world, and what we don't like in the world.

The instinct to care for our young is also part of the limbic system. This amazing extra 'app' evolved in the brain so that mammals and birds could nurture and protect their young, thus enabling better survival of the species – an evolutionary leap forwards. Lionesses protect their young ferociously. They even work together to fight and chase away male lions who threaten their cubs. Birds, too, go to great lengths to feed and protect their young. Some species of penguins dive off rocky cliffs into stormy seas in order to bring back fish for their young, returning bloody and battered from each voyage. A few years ago, when walking across the moors in North Uist, I nearly trod on a nest of Golden Plover chicks. Their mother had left the nest on my approach, making a great noise in order to distract me and draw me away from her chicks. She was ready to offer herself as prey rather than have her chicks endangered. I was trying so hard to keep a wide berth of her and her chicks that I nearly trod on the deserted open nest. The chicks were both silent and perfectly camouflaged. Never has my foot in its heavy grey climbing boot looked so Godzilla-like as I suddenly saw the precious chicks and hopped to one side.

Evolution did not stop at the limbic system. The amazing cerebral neocortex (meaning 'new bark' in Latin) began its remarkable expansion in the mammalian brain only two to three million years ago. The neocortex is the part of the brain nearest the skull, the part that looks like a walnut, full of deep indentations and grooves. It is suggested that the neocortex grew and increased in size in our ancestors in response to pressures for greater cooperation and social harmony. It enables complex language and reasoning processes. Interestingly, the mammal with the greatest number of neocortical nerve cells is that most playful of creatures, the dolphin. The neocortex is the newest, most evolved part of the brain, a part we do not yet fully understand.

Our human brains therefore possess the original reptilian

program plus two major upgrades – the amazing iHuman3.
Who would want to settle for Reptilian1? If we think of it
in mobile phone terms, there's no competition: we want the
upgrades and we want to make full use of all the fascinating
new apps. But if, despite having the upgrade, we think only
from the point of view of the reptilian brain, then all this
'we' thinking, all this nurture and care for the next generation puts 'me' as an individual at risk and is highly suspect.
This neocortex capacity for compassion and forgiveness of
enemies looks like plain suicide from the point of view
of our ancient, reptilian brain, the part that has helped
us survive thus far. Surely that ancestral part of our brain
deserves our loyalty, especially when it often calls with such
urgency? Hadn't we better listen to the reptilian brain and
limbic system with their dire warnings of enemies, and
maybe arm ourselves a bit better, be a little less trusting of
man's innate goodness? Better safe than sorry, after all.

The problem is that our highly evolved neocortex,
obedient to the anxious urgings of our old reptilian brain,
is now able to construct highly evolved weaponry – but
our reptilian brain and limbic system do not know that we
have upgraded from caveman's club to nuclear missile. They
do not know that the destructive power of present-day
weaponry can no longer keep any user of such weapons
safe. Ecologists and nuclear physicists agree that, given the
phenomenally destructive and polluting power of present-
day nuclear weapons, any outbreak of nuclear hostilities
in either hemisphere would be followed by catastrophic
climate change, crop failure, starvation and radioactive
pollution across the globe. We now have weapons that
we literally cannot use without endangering not only the

survival of our own species, but all other species too … with the possible exception of the cockroach. We know these weapons are unusable and yet, spurred on by the fear that our enemies may have bigger missiles up their sleeves, we continue to invent and build bigger and still more destructive weapons.

'Better safe than sorry' was appropriate when it just meant 'Remember to take the hunting club with you when you leave the cave.' It no longer applies to a nuclear arms race that has spun out of control in a world where we will all be *unsafe* and desperately sorry if we ever fire one of these weapons at another country. Albert Einstein said in 1946, 'The unleashed power of the atom has changed everything save our modes of thinking and we thus drift towards unparalleled catastrophe.' [6]

Can we evolve and urgently change our 'mode of thinking'? The future of our children depends on which view we choose to live by, whether we evolve and adopt the 'we' view – take the risk of trusting man's innate goodness and choose to build together a cooperative, inclusive world based on trust in our greater possibilities, a world where 'our humanity exceeds our technology' – or whether we persist in a 'me against them' view – the aggressive/defensive individualistic view, a world where global issues are of concern only when they strongly impact on me and my country, a world that believes nuclear weapons are a necessity for survival, a world that helplessly 'drifts towards unparalleled catastrophe'. The choice of which world view we opt for, and therefore which world we create for our children, has never been more urgent. As Martin Luther King Jr said, 'We must learn to live together as brothers or perish together as fools.' [7]

What Increases Our Suffering and Lessens Our Happiness?

We are capable of so much more brother-and-sisterhood than we presently believe possible. Our reptilian brain cannot trust – it was built not to trust, it was built to react and to get us out of danger. It isn't wrong or bad, and neither is our limbic system. Both are a natural and essential part of us. 'Better safe than sorry' is the only message they can give. But it is not the only message our cerebral neocortex has to listen to. Our neocortex has wider possibilities, is rich in greater, more inclusive responses that embrace all of humanity.

What is our own view? Do we agree with the Dalai Lama that adopting an inclusive 'we' attitude is simple common sense, or does our fearfulness keep us wedded to a more primitive 'me versus you' view of the world?

We travel much lighter when we adopt the 'we' view. Despite the apparent prevalence of the 'me/you' view in the world today, we also often function from the 'we' view. We certainly aspire to it. Why else would we so admire heroes and heroines who risk their lives for others? Why would we give so generously to help victims of a natural disaster if we did not also see them as 'us'? Why do parents, and many a stranger too, put their own lives at risk as they instantly rush to pull a child out of the way of an oncoming car? I was a rural GP who attended many road traffic accidents, and I have seen how passers-by behave. You only get the very occasional voyeur. Nearly all the folk who stop are desperate to help the injured one; will hold a stranger's head for half an hour until the ambulance arrives so that his spinal cord is protected, will look after a frightened child, will put themselves at risk without thinking. People's automatic reactions can be extraordinarily generous and selfless.

The neuroscientist Richard Davidson suggests that compassion and kindness, just like language, are human potentials present within each one of us when we are born. However, we develop and express these potentials only if they are demonstrated by the adults nurturing us. Feral children who never hear a spoken word do not learn to speak. Language only develops in a 'speaking environment'. Davidson suggests that, just as with language, we can only develop and fully express the compassion innate in us if we ourselves are brought up in a compassionate environment. [8]

Neuroscientists tell us that we currently utilise only a tiny part of our complex brains. We have more capacity than we think we do. We do not have to lead our lives according to the frightened urgings of a small and primitive part of our brain. We can start to become familiar with greater possibilities within our brain and within ourselves. We are capable of so much more and, extraordinarily, even one individual developing a wider vision, a more inclusive response, can have immeasurable consequences for the whole world. Mahatma Gandhi and Martin Luther King Jr demonstrated this.

So did Nelson Mandela.

Out of Africa

Nelson Mandela spent twenty-seven years imprisoned in South Africa. During his incarceration on Robben Island, his son died, his daughters grew up, his wife was treated brutally by the apartheid regime and his people were murdered. He had every reason to come out of jail embittered and full of hatred. He had every reason to give up all hope of there being any goodness in man, any joy in life. Yet throughout his years on Robben Island he continued to believe in the fundamental power of love over hatred. He wrote, 'People must learn to hate, and if they can learn to hate, they can be taught to love, for love comes more naturally to the human heart than its opposite.' Even at his lowest ebb, he was able to see the occasional flash of humanity in a prison guard, and that was enough to reassure him. [9]

Based on his wonderfully generous take on life, Mandela was able to forgive his gaolers and forgive those who enforced the misery of apartheid on his people for over forty years. He was therefore able to negotiate with de Klerk in 1990 from a position of great clarity and strength, since he himself was uncluttered by hatred. His remarkable stature at the time of independence in 1994, saved South Africa from the fearful bloodbath that most had predicted. Warring factions (both white on black, and black on black) followed his leadership and literally laid down their arms. He told them, 'We can't win a war. But we can win an election.'

Proof that there is nothing powerless about an unwavering belief in human kindness, nothing weak in the power of forgiveness. Forgiveness and love can apparently move mountains of hatred, as Mandela's life demonstrated. Love in a time of fear is not a naive pipedream. When lived, it is one of the most powerful forces on the planet.

Is our own take on life less inclusive and forgiving than Mandela's? I sense that mine is. When I watch the news it can seem that the world is very different, that it is red in tooth and claw. We can get the impression that we must always strive to get to the top, and even there can never be safe because of rivals baying at our heels. In such a competitive, hostile world any insult requires revenge, any loss must be instantly recouped, any mistake punished and all signs of personal vulnerability rapidly hidden. In such a world, kindness is portrayed as weakness, forgiveness as a mental aberration. Even the softer ties of love within the family become infected by the pervading fear and insecurity: *If I must be the strongest then my spouse must be the most attractive, my children the most successful, my house the most impressive and my bank balance the one with the most zeroes. I must constantly make deals that secure my position at the top. I must crush my competitors or they will crush me. My very survival depends on my ability to outwit and outperform others . . . if I believe that view.*

Which of these two world views – the highly evolved 'we' view, or the more primitive 'me against them' view – do we ourselves believe? Which of these two worlds do we create and then inhabit? For the moment, our global structures all seem to be premised on the latter view. Our economy is based on an overriding profit motive that drives relentless competition and insists on the imperative of continual growth. Ensuing need and greed drive a frenetic work pace. Those at the top award themselves ever-bigger bonuses while those at the bottom have little chance of moving upwards, and find their scant resources squeezed. We cease to be able to communicate or listen to each other in such a world. The pace at which the rich are getting richer accelerates further. Within our society a massive income gap yawns between rich and poor. The wealthy live with their equally rich friends in their seemingly luxurious wealth-bubble, the poor live with others of similarly low incomes in their own much drabber bubble. Anyone who suggests that businesses should be less profit-driven and should show concern for their whole workforce, not just the select few who make it to the top, is viewed as naive and is told, 'Look, that's just not how the world is.'

Are any of us free in such a world? Are even the one per cent at the top of the wealth pyramid – who now own as much as the rest of the world put together and whose lifestyles defy the imagination of the rest of us – are they really free? Or are they still trapped, competing with each other, competing with their own bank balances? The sheer futility of all that concentrated effort when, as they say in Scotland, 'There are nae pockets in a shroud.' A story is told of two gentlemen at a wealthy friend's funeral. As they walk away from the graveside one says to the other, 'How much did he leave, I wonder?' The other answers, 'Oh, I think everything.'

Once, when on holiday in Malta, we were ferried across the Grand Harbour in Valletta by a toothless, elderly boatman in an equally elderly wooden boat. My daughter and I gawped in amazement as a yacht the size of a Holiday Inn hove into view, dwarfing all around it. Our boatman grinned and said, 'Abramovich – his smaller yacht.' As we shook our heads in amazement, the boatman laughed again and said, gesturing to himself and then the yacht, 'Me and Abramovich, ten feet under – same, same!' Huge grin. His take on life freed him from envy, and helped us to see more clearly too.

How did the rich become so rich? Did they generate their wealth by creating new technologies? In a few cases, yes, but the majority of the richest people in the world got there by redistributing the world's existing wealth into their own bank balances. They robbed a lot of Pauls to pay their very own Peter. The richest sixty-two people in the world now own as much as the poorer half of the world's population. This means that the sixty-two richest billionaires in the world presently own as much wealth as the 3.6 billion poorest people. [10] Worse, this combined wealth of the richest sixty-two people has increased by more than half-a-trillion dollars since 2010, while the wealth of the poorest half of the world's population has fallen by over a trillion dollars in the same period. When wealth distribution in society has become this far out of kilter, nobody is truly free, and society is deeply unstable.

Nelson Mandela knew that freedom for all depends on social justice for all. He saw that social injustice robs both the oppressor and the oppressed of their common humanity. He wrote from his prison cell, 'the oppressor must be liberated just as surely as the oppressed ... I am not truly free if I am taking away someone else's freedom, just as surely as I am not free when my freedom is taken from me.' [11]

So if fear, fixity, fury and foolishness are the inner seeds, or tendencies, within us that greatly add to our suffering, and indeed threaten our future, what are the seeds or qualities within us that nourish our happiness, lessen our suffering and lighten our lives? What are the seeds within us that we need to water and cultivate in order to survive and thrive?

Four

What Lessens Our Suffering and Increases Our Happiness?

The Dalai Lama's answer to this question is clear. He describes how we all strive to avoid physical pain. We seek to cure diseases and build up our physical immunity. He goes on to say, 'Mental pain is equally bad, so we should try to alleviate it as well. The way to do this is to develop mental immunity ... Mental immunity is just learning to avoid the destructive emotions, and to develop the positive ones.'[1]

What, then are the positive emotions we should practise?

Kindness
Interestingly, and topically, the word 'kind' has the same derivation as the word 'kin'. They both come from the Old English *cynde/gecynde*, meaning 'natural, native or with the feeling that relatives have for each other'. As if confirming the derivation of the English word, the Dalai Lama, who states that his religion is kindness, says that wherever he goes in the world he meets human beings who, just like him,

wish to be happy and avoid suffering. He says he has never yet met a stranger, in all his travels. My son understood this as a teenager when he read Primo Levi's writings on the nightmare of life in World War Two concentration camps. Adam looked at me and said, 'You have to believe the other person is completely different from you before you can treat them that way, don't you?' When we recognise that the other person is just like us, kindness happens naturally. Kindness has that quality of kinship, of family, to it. Cruelty does not.

Again, we need to check our underlying beliefs. Do we believe that human beings are generally untrustworthy and only out for Number One, or do we trust that fundamentally the human heart is kind? It is important that we check our view again and again, as our view 'pre-orders' reality and determines which positive teachings – if any – we can take in and act upon.

In the Buddhist understanding, fundamental human nature is like a diamond covered in mud. The diamond of goodness and purity is there in all beings and can never be altered, but it is often covered over with mud so that it cannot be seen. We can even forget it is there, but it is, and is equally pure in all of us. It is the same goodness whether we are saint or sinner. Simply, the saints have found their hidden treasure and are manifesting its goodness. Unless we begin to see what it was that Mandela saw – the underlying goodness in others – we can never lay down our weapons. We can never trust and be kind to ourselves and to others.

I can think of so many times when kindness has been shown to me in my life. A very simple one that stands out was during my time as a dormitory helper at the Camphill Community in Aberdeen. I was a tired twenty-four-year-old and had been asked to stand in for a fellow volunteer who was sick. It was my one day off in a busy week and I was not in the most generous of moods. The three girls aged around seven who I had been asked to look after were not keen on getting ready for the walk I had suggested. They played games around me. Socks and shoes started to be thrown across the room. I suddenly lost it. I shouted at them, told them to get ready 'Now!' in my angriest voice – and was immediately crushed by their frightened obedience. I was further crushed by the senior house-mother coming quietly into the dormitory. She had heard the temper in my voice, probably from several rooms away. I felt small and ashamed, expecting a telling-off myself in turn. Yet without a hint of a frown she beamed at me while calmly helping the children with their coats. We all chatted gently about where we were walking to and then she warmly waved us off. She simply came in and was equally kind to all of us. It was quietly done.

Kindness alters how we experience things. My daughter, a nurse, was working in a busy surgical ward. One of her patients had just come back from major surgery, fully conscious but in a fair degree of pain. It took a while for the team to get his pain relief right. As my daughter finished her shift she apologised to the patient, saying, 'I'm so sorry we didn't relieve your pain more quickly.' The man smiled at her and replied, 'Don't worry. Your kindness and concern halved the pain in the first place.'

Acceptance

Acceptance is an active process. It is neither passive nor resigned. It takes maturity to let everything be, just as it is, while being aware of our own emotions inside as well as external events outside. Only then we can respond in full awareness. Acceptance is not acquiescence. True acceptance is an opportunity to then be creative. Whatever the situation, we can work with it better when we stop rebelling against it, manipulating it, or trying to pretend it is other than it is. Once we let all information in, without prior prejudice, we are able to take whatever action is most appropriate. Like Mandela, we can act with power from a calmer, less reactive place.

Tolerance

We can exercise tolerance only by letting in that which we experience as different from us, that which is difficult for us, that which challenges us. Otherwise we are simply living in a comfortable bubble with like-minded friends while fondly imagining ourselves to be tolerant.

I became a university student in heady times. My first year in Edinburgh saw students marching down Princes Street waving banners emblazoned with the tolerant message 'Disembowel Enoch Powell'. It had a certain ring to it, and someone had unwisely suggested him as university rector. I smoked marijuana *and* inhaled. I floated around hospital wards in long skirts, eye-to-eye with consultants in my two-inch platform shoes. I became an ardent feminist, even joining a clearly upwardly-mobile 'consciousness-raising group' – a group that left my own state of consciousness firmly unrisen. I loved my time at university and found wonderful, like-minded friends. I even married one! I was so lucky, but quite unaware of the protected, like-minded bubble that I lived in at that time. I think I just thought I had good fortune and remarkably good taste . . .

When the realities of other peoples' very different views impacted on me, I knew my stance and reacted firmly. At my first junior doctor interview, in 1976, one of the two male consultants asked me in somewhat bored tones, 'And tell me, Miss Gunn, *if* you were to get married,' – it was a six-month post I was applying for – 'do you think that your marriage would affect your medical career?' I was outraged and decided the job could go hang. I responded, 'I certainly hope so. It wouldn't be much of a marriage if it didn't affect my medical career. Hasn't your marriage affected yours?' The other consultant found this so funny that I wondered whether I might still have a chance of the job.

John and I went out to Malawi as young idealists hoping to do our best working in the government hospitals there. On arrival we had a three-month orientation period at the 800-bed main hospital in the capital at the time, Blantyre. At night you were the only doctor on for the entire hospital. A stuttering tannoy system informed you which ward next needed you urgently. When we arrived at the hospital, the Malawian medical superintendent Dr Mukandawire, shook my newly married hand and asked how hospital staff should differentiate between me and John. I explained that was no problem: I had kept my maiden name and could be addressed as Dr Gunn. Dr Mukandawire beamed, shook his head at the complete nonsense of this and said, 'Ah, no. *You* will be known as Dr Mrs Gills.' (My husband's surname, or near cousin to it.) '*He* will be known as Dr Mr Gills.' To have objected would have appeared racist. It's damnable when two dearly held righteousnesses conflict. My feminism swallowed hard and for the next three years I answered to the title of 'Dr Mrs Jill', a lesson in humility and tolerance if ever there was one.

We were then sent to a district hospital on the Mozambique border. There was a very small expatriate community in the area, largely formed of missionary sisters and priests from Europe. The only other white couple in the area greeted our arrival with enthusiasm, an enthusiasm only slightly muted by our dismal inability to play bridge. Their names were Richard and Jane. They were in their seventies and they were delightful. Jane helped me plant my new garden, advising me to replant the tree I had put too close to our kitchen wall, telling me how often to water, endlessly bringing cuttings from her own garden. Together we watched our garden grow in what seemed like minutes.

Richard and Jane were white Rhodesians through and through. When talk of the recent Rhodesian war came up, I realised Richard had not only fought in it but had also firmly supported white Rhodesian dominance. He was now an exile from the new Zimbabwe, from the country he so loved, had grown up in, farmed in and lost his fortune in. He now had to continue farming in another country well into his late seventies. It was clear he could never leave Africa; Africa was in his blood. Yet I was shocked by his high-handed manner with local Malawian workers. I had never seen someone I considered my friend act so rudely to people of different colour. It really challenged me.

Richard and Jane wanted to come and see round the newly built hospital we had just moved into. We arranged a day. John was in theatre when I showed them round our four wards. At each ward our wonderful, smartly dressed Malawian nurses and clinical officers leapt to their feet, beaming with joy to meet visitors, and shook hands enthusiastically with both Richard and Jane as I introduced everyone by name. I commented to John later that evening that both Richard and Jane had looked pretty shaken by the end of the visit. I berated myself for pointing out all the severely malnourished children we then had in the ward. I realised it had probably been too much suffering, all at once, for their unaccustomed eyes.

John answered, 'Yes; they might have looked pale because of that. But I think it would also have been a great shock to them to shake so many black hands in one afternoon.' This turned out to be true. So our way of being with Malawians had in turn challenged Richard and Jane's ways. We learned from each other as we tolerated each other's differences. We spoke of our differences and remained friends. Size helped. In a larger community we might each have dismissed the other on first meeting. Malawi taught us so much about tolerance, in every way.

Humility and humour

You know the way the Dalai Lama walks on to a stage, slightly stooped, bowing and waving to the audience, acknowledging everyone else, completely at ease? He seems the embodiment of humility, warmth and humour. The Dalai Lama said that when he first had to address a large gathering as a young man, he felt very nervous until he realised that there really was nothing to be intimidated by. He said to himself, 'These people are all human beings just like me. There is no difference between us.' [2] Since then he has avoided all formality and remains at ease wherever he goes, knowing that he is simply meeting others just like him.

Well

A friend said to me, 'You know these Buddhist masters, they all have the same sort of warm, easy smile, they are always ready to see the funny side of anything ridiculous in life, they never take themselves too seriously – while treating the teachings they give with utter seriousness and respect.' Again and again, the teachers emphasise to us the importance of humility, of our not being the upturned pot, full of pride, into which no teachings can be poured. Humility and humour go together; it's so much easier to be humble when you've just had a belly-laugh at your own ridiculousness. In Tibet they say that wisdom, just like humility, gathers in the low places, the valleys, and they add, 'And where does spring happen first?' Again, down in the valleys.

In Malawi I was in charge of a 100-bed paediatric ward that was often full of severely malnourished children. I was heartbroken by the stick-like limbs of these children, their suffering, their abject misery. Their cries filled our ears as we fed them, treated their infections, dressed their wounds, joyfully watched them gain weight or sadly watched them die. I noticed that the minute a child showed the slightest sign of recovery (usually hinted at by the first shy return of a smile to their young face) the mother, who always stayed to care for her child in hospital, would say she had to take the child home now. I would beg and plead with her to wait a week longer, let the child at least gain some more weight before returning to a distant village. I knew what danger the child was still in – one untreated bout of malaria could be fatal. The mother would smile, seemingly acquiesce, then disappear during the night with her child. '*Anatawa* – she has absconded – doctor,' the nurses would tell me in the morning with a shake of their heads.

I honed my Chichewa and began lecturing all mothers of malnourished babies on how vital it was that they stayed in the ward long enough for their child to recover. I was on a mission. The mothers would courteously listen to this righteous, white-skinned mother of none, and continue to leave in the night as soon as a glint of improvement appeared in their child. I despaired of Malawian mothers.

Then I started doing weekly visits to our faraway rural health clinics. We would go to villages, hang our weighing scales from a sturdy branch and weigh all the children under five years old. I saw how all the work of tilling the fields, sowing the maize and ensuring next year's food supply fell to the women. I realised that any mother, no matter how much she loved her malnourished toddler on the ward, could spare only so much time from crop-tending this year, or *all* her children would starve the next year. When the mother quietly said, 'I must take the child home now,' she said it because it was the truth. When I saw this, I stopped berating the mothers. I saw I was mistaken in my righteous judgments. I sent those I had lectured my mute, and humble, apologies.

Fast-forward to 2011 for an event full of humour as well as humility. The humour was all on Lama Yeshe's part; the humility came – reluctantly – from me. I was one year into my cancer recurrence. The mass was slowly shrinking, but between scans I had no idea what it was doing. I felt very pessimistic about surviving longer than a few years. John, on the other hand, had just taken over a demanding new job in central Edinburgh, arranged before I got ill. He was often away on business, and even when he was home I felt he was often away on business in his head. Adam and

Rebecca were away leading their own lives. I had resigned my GP job, too tired to continue, two years previously and I felt pretty defunct. Our dog Tessa had just died and I really missed her geriatric, gently snoring presence in the kitchen. I was feeling bereft and sorry for myself. Meeting with Lama Yeshe, I complained (never a wise thing to do when talking to a Tibetan lama) that my husband was often away with his new job and that at times I felt left behind and abandoned.

Lama Yeshe was having none of it. His response was instant. His arm moved with an authoritative sweep – of all that I had just said – in the direction of the window as he said, 'That is *very* childish thinking.'

It was such an unexpectedly blunt response that I burst out laughing. 'Lama Yeshe, I *know* it's childish thinking. I'm embarrassed and ashamed to be admitting it to you.'

At which, Lama Yeshe's arm swept towards the window again as he said, 'Oh, you Westerners and your guilt and shame. That can go, too.' (And go it did, out the window.)

There was nothing left in the room to discuss. Once again I had gone in heavy, taking myself and my situation very seriously, and come out light – and laughing.

Compassion, self-compassion and forgiveness
Compassion is such a vast, limitless energy. While empathy is the ability to pick up the feelings of another person, compassion contains something more. Compassion is the sensing and deep feeling of another's suffering accompanied by the strong wish to ease that suffering.

The Dalai Lama says that, having spoken with many scientists, teachers, activists and healthcare professionals from around the world, 'it is clear that the only way to truly change the world is through teaching compassion ... too much self-centred thinking is the source of suffering ... even scientists now say basic human nature is compassionate.'[3]

Chöje Akong Rinpoche, Lama Yeshe's older brother and founder of Samye Ling Tibetan Buddhist monastery in Scotland, was the deepest embodiment of compassion. In the 1950s, Akong Rinpoche was a young, highly venerated lama in Tibet. Escaping from the invading Chinese, he lost his monastery, his family and his country. He, Lama Yeshe and another high lama, Chögyam Trungpa, arrived in India in 1960 after a gruelling ten-month journey. Travelling with a large group of Tibetan refugees, they had struggled through mountain passes, icy swollen rivers, starvation, exhaustion, hypothermia and, on several occasions, Chinese bullets. Of the original group of 300 refugees, only thirteen made it to India.

From India, Akong Rinpoche travelled to Britain, and to Oxford. There he worked as a hospital porter, earning money while Chögyam Trungpa studied at the university. And so Oxford patients were pushed to theatre by a Tibetan high lama who until recently had been treated with immense respect by all, was accustomed to riding on horseback, rarely walking far, and used to being looked after by a host of attendants. Now he was a porter in a busy NHS hospital, a foreign refugee with little English who had never pushed a trolley before in his life. Ward staff impatiently admonished him for taking too long, so he speeded up. Fellow porters then ordered him to slow down or they would lose their jobs. He said those were the years when he really worked on his mind.

In 1967, he and Chögyam Trungpa founded Samye Ling Tibetan Buddhist monastery in Scotland. Chögyam Trungpa later moved on to the US to teach. Akong Rinpoche nurtured the growing community and oversaw the building of the temple. He developed Tara Rokpa Therapy to help relieve the suffering he observed in so many visitors. He started Buddhist centres in many British and European cities, and then went on to found the world-wide charity ROKPA to help those in need in Nepal, the Tibet Autonomous Region, Zimbabwe and South Africa. He said that in 1959, when he and his fellow travellers were starving during their flight from Tibet, he vowed that if he survived he would feed those who were hungry. He never stopped working for others and never judged or turned away those in need of help. He initiated and supervised the work of each of these international projects, making gruelling annual trips to visit them. He worked tirelessly for the good of others in Scotland and across the world.

I was overawed when I first encountered Akong Rinpoche in the 1990s. He was seated on a silk-bedecked throne in the Samye Ling temple, clad in brightly brocaded robes, giving teachings. (I later learned that he was as often to be found in workman's clothes, wielding a spade or builder's trowel. Indeed, when the Samye Ling sewage system seized up, it was Akong Rinpoche who was first down the hole to sort out the problem.) The temple was filled with hundreds of students bowing to him. Everyone listened in deeply respectful silence when he spoke. I had never seen someone being treated with quite such reverence and love by so many. He was teaching on compassion. He described how in the West we often lack self-compassion.

Our culture teaches us to be highly self-critical. As a result we instantly beat ourselves up whenever we see that we've made a mistake. He questioned our underlying assumption that we should somehow be capable of avoiding making mistakes. He used his own life as an example:

'All my life I have made mistakes. And I will go on making mistakes – not because I wish to, simply because I lack the wisdom to avoid them. The only stupidity is to continue to make the same mistake. Once we see we have made a mistake, regret and vow not to make that mistake again. So I ask all of you from now on: only make new mistakes!'

I had never heard anything quite like this before. A man clearly so wise, so massively respected, sitting on a throne in a temple and not only admitting to a large audience that he had made mistakes his whole life long, but also admitting that he remained liable to continue doing so. His humility took my breath away. And what he said made complete sense. I was changed by his teaching and by his presence. It was impossible not to be.

Akong Rinpoche's advice always comes to my aid when I slip into the old default mode of beating myself up for doing something wrong. His effortless forgiveness reminds me yet again to release the old blame habit. As your gaze widens with regular meditation and mindfulness, you begin to see, quite clearly – and painfully – how you have generated a lot of your own and others' suffering in the past, mainly due to a certain unseen fixity of reaction. Seeing this is rather like going through the mincer. It is certainly bracing. A kindly eye is all. Unless you can forgive yourself, as well as the other, you can hardly bear to look. Remembering Akong Rinpoche's teaching on the making of mistakes always helps me to forgive all past mistakes in myself or anyone else and just come back to the present moment – to be here, now.

In 2013 Akong Rinpoche was tragically murdered while supervising and funding ROKPA projects in the Tibetan region of China. A Chinese court pronounced the death penalty on his two killers, but Rinpoche's family and Samye Ling pleaded for clemency. Rinpoche's eldest son, Jigme Tarap, asked friends and students to show compassion to the convicted men, saying that he can never forget his father telling him: 'If you forget everything I say, remember not to forget: the greatest power is compassion.'

Lama Yeshe wrote in an open letter to the community:

When I learnt of the circumstances of my brother's death and the identities of those who killed him and his nephew and driver, I felt extremely sorry for them because it shows how one moment of misguided anger can ruin so many lives. So instead of feeling angry, I feel compassion for them and think about how much bad karma these misguided persons have created for themselves and others. I would like to let our friends, who wish to do something for my brother and me, know that this is the time for forgiveness . . . I have been able to forgive and this is how I was freed from my suffering. I urge you to keep a compassionate and positive mind, and let us now work together to continue Rinpoche's activity.

And that is what the Samye Ling community, led by Lama Yeshe, has done. Lama Yeshe's commitment, presence and joyfulness continues undimmed. I have never seen the power of forgiveness evidenced so deeply.

Appreciation, gratitude and generosity

When I lived in rural Africa, I appreciated so much what I

had there. I was treating starving children in the hospital so I appreciated my own food, and I appreciated the generosity of the donors who supplied all the precious dried milk we fed the children. I kept seeing others so much less fortunate than me in every way. I could only work hard, and never fail to appreciate all the material security and freedom that I had in comparison. It was staring me in the face.

The roads we trundled over in our bone-shaking hospital Land Rover to get to our scattered health centres would become deeply pot-holed in the rainy season. They became more riverbed than road. I really appreciated their sudden return to smoothness, once they had been levelled again by the grading lorry at the start of the dry season. In the shops, goods were so often 'temporarily' out of stock (in reality this meant months) that you really appreciated a toilet roll when you found one again. A phone call home was so tricky to arrange that I really appreciated my mother's voice on the line the few times that all the tenuous connections managed to stay together.

Then I came back to Britain. Within weeks I had stopped appreciating all the everyday occurrences that had given me joy in Africa because now I expected them. In the same way, although I would have said that working as a doctor I always appreciated my own good health, I didn't really appreciate it. Not until it wasn't there any more. Then, especially after the recurrence of my cancer, I started really appreciating being alive. After initially experiencing such terror, and then such ongoing release from terror, all I can ever do when I meet Lama Yeshe is to tell him how grateful I am for his help. He answers, 'Good. Now you will never be poor again. Now you have the practice of gratitude.'

All the Buddhist teachers emphasise the importance of practising generosity. At first I interpreted this according to my old understanding: 'You're right. I've got so much more than so many others in the world. Poor them. I really should do more, give away more of my income in order to help others.' It took me a while to get a feel for the fact that generosity is really about letting go of your own contracted sense of self and loosening up. Including others and giving to them is in fact a way of enlarging your own tight world. It is the giver who genuinely benefits by *giving away* instead of *grasping towards*.

There is a Buddhist story about a rich man who confessed to the Buddha that generosity was the one practice he found almost impossible (echoing the New Testament parable about the difficulties of a rich man entering the kingdom of heaven). The Buddha asked this man to quietly practise placing something precious in his right hand, then give it to his left hand, then give it back to his right hand and to continue with this practice. Gradually, over time, he was able to pass the precious object from his own hand into another's hand. I love the way we are encouraged to start from where we are and gently work from there, patiently, persistently.

Patience and perseverance

Working in the NHS means that you become accustomed to a wide variety of human behaviour. I got used to defusing angry situations and working with upset people. All in all, I thought I was a pretty patient and tolerant human being. Then I read the Buddhist definition of patience: 'Patience – bearing no anger against anyone.' Good heavens, I'd never thought of patience as meaning *that*.

What I had been calling patience was in fact 'me carrying on being nice' despite a whole heap of suppressed irritation inside me. I could see that the practice of patience would actually be effortless if there were no anger to hold back in the first place. Anger is often based on righteous judgments about others. Old habits die hard. I am still working on not judging so much in the first place, but at least I have a notion of a direction of travel regarding patience. It is not that we have to tolerate intolerable behaviour. We do not, and we should act firmly to protect ourselves against it. It's just that we don't need to burn ourselves up with angry judgments along the way, such as (in my own case): 'He should not be acting like this' (*well, he is*); 'I should not have to put up with this sort of thing' (*you don't have to – take action*); 'She should not be shouting' (*again, she already is. Deal with it appropriately*); and so on. Intrigued by the effortlessness of true patience, and seeing it in others, helps me to slowly drop my old way – of being impatient.

To me, persevering meant putting your shoulder to the wheel and working hard, putting in strenuous ongoing effort, and feeling bad when you sloped off or slackened. I get bored quite easily. I viewed perseverance as one of those burdensome things I wasn't much good at.

So why, then, did the Buddhist teachings describe perseverance (or diligence) as 'joyful effort'? Ringu Tulku Rinpoche, another great Tibetan teacher, helped me by describing joyful effort as being similar to the type of effort we Westerners apply to our hobbies, to the pastimes we enjoy and choose. I enjoy sewing and can work late into the night finishing a garment. It doesn't feel like work at all. I don't even notice how much time has passed doing it. I felt the same when I went on a skiing week and had learned how to descend the slopes without falling over. I couldn't wait to get back on the ski tow and give it another try. That didn't feel like perseverance. It was pure enthusiasm and enjoyment *because it was what I wanted to do*.

I realised that I had been using 'perseverance' to describe the effort involved in doing something that deep down I didn't really want to do. That puts a lot of resistance, plus extra effort to overcome that resistance, into the process. However, if I looked deeply and decided *Yes, for me this is worthwhile and I actually want to do this* – be it about meditation practice or any other activity – then easy, joyful effort (almost effortlessness) moved into the process.

Five

What Tools Do We Need to Effect These Changes?

The Guest House
This being human is a guest house.
Every morning a new arrival.

A joy, a depression, a meanness,
some momentary awareness comes
as an unexpected visitor.

Welcome and entertain them all!
Even if they're a crowd of sorrows,
who violently sweep your house
empty of its furniture,
still, treat each guest honourably.
He may be clearing you out
for some new delight.

The dark thought, the shame, the malice,
meet them at the door laughing,
and invite them in.

Well

Be grateful for whoever comes,
because each has been sent
as a guide from beyond. [1]

Jalāl ad-Dīn Muhammad Rūmī
(translated by Coleman Barks)

Spaciousness, openness and a new kind of not-knowing became the qualities I valued when illness came into my life. Priorities shifted. What mattered were family and friends. What mattered was not missing the moments of good health, the happy moments, as I could make no assumptions as to how the next moment would be. I knew this so clearly I was surprised that I hadn't always known this, because of course it had applied to 'healthy me' all along. It applies to us all in every moment. None of us know what the next moment will bring.

I relished the good times with new joy. It seemed natural to want to make them last, to continue. But I found that if I clung to the good moments they weren't quite so good. Whenever I held on to happiness, an anxiety had already entered in; the next possibly 'bad' moment was intruding on the happy present. I realised that openness meant just that – being equally open to all that life would bring: the good, the bad, and the ugly too. I liked Rumi's advice to 'treat each guest honourably'. I liked the novel thought of greeting my own shame or even malice 'at the door laughing'. Rumi's poems helped me to learn new ways of meeting this unexpectedness that had erupted in my life, of allowing it all while somehow staying present, staying hospitable to all that was happening. Attending weekend courses on mindfulness and yoga helped too. I noticed that when my thoughts went one way I could be very frightened. When they went another way I could be quite steady. I wanted to know more about what determined my inner weather. Clearly it was affected by external events, but it was ultimately determined by *how I chose to respond* to those events.

Everything we do or say begins first in our mind as a thought, an idea, an intention. Man had to *want* to go to the moon before he set about finding ways of building a rocket to get him there. I became a doctor on the whim of my twelve-year-old self, but where did that whim come from? I travelled to work in Africa because I felt drawn there. I began writing this book because I had an urge to do so, and hoped others might be interested to read it. What makes us think the way we do? If we understand that, then we are much closer to understanding what makes us act the way we do. An Indian proverb states that going out to sort the world without first coming to terms with your own inner conflicts is rather like 'going out to follow the tracks in the jungle while the elephant you are looking for is rampaging in your own house'.

It is such an adventure, stopping and observing the workings of our own mind. We know a lot about the terrain out there (the world), we know a lot about the workings of the vehicle in which we move through the world (our body) but we are often not that well acquainted with the one who is driving the vehicle – our own mind. To simply stop and pay attention both to what is happening outside us and to what is happening within us, moment by moment, can be shocking, humbling, illuminating and freeing. I've always loved exploring and travelling. When I became unwell my exploring initially felt hobbled, even ended. For a while I mourned the trekking holidays I had planned for the future, those expeditions to parts of the world that I'd never seen. Then I began to realise that now was time for a different type of discovery. Time to be still, let be, become more aware of what was happening right here, right now. Anyone can do this, any time, in any state of health. No one is excluded.

In the West our explorations have been adventurous and wide-reaching. They have tended to be out there, into the world. Empires were built following the explorations of Vasco de Gama, Christopher Columbus, Captain Cook and so many others. We didn't know what lands lay across the sea from us, we wanted to know, and so we set sail to find out. Initially the maps marked unknown territories as 'There be dragons', but gradually the unknown territories became named, walked on, included in our reassuring global maps of the known. These lands had of course been very well known to their own native inhabitants long before anyone from Europe 'discovered' them, but we all see life from our own culture's perspective. Having named and tried to own most of the land we found, we then started exploring the nature of life, making remarkable discoveries in science and technology. We are naturally curious, always wanting to know more.

Medical science explored the human body and we now understand how our hearts, lungs, kidneys, livers, metabolism and neurons function, an Aladdin's cave of knowledge and expertise allowing old organs to be replaced with new. Freud and Jung made great breakthroughs in understanding the 'diseased' human mind, but in general in Western culture no great emphasis was placed on each person gently befriending his or her own mind and taking responsibility for understanding it. As a culture we remained oddly disinterested in what makes our mind – the discoverer (and wielder) of all this amazing knowledge – tick. Our consumerist culture tends to draw our attention ever outwards, looking in the direction of all that is still to be discovered *out there*, of all that is yet to be purchased.

In contrast, many Eastern cultures placed more of an emphasis on investigating and understanding the human mind – not as an external object 'out there' but as an individual and intimate investigation of 'in here'. This is a very different type of exploration. My first meditation teacher explained that 'meditation is simply getting to know your own mind'. The Tibetan word for meditation, *gom*, means familiarisation (with our own mind). Our mind is extremely powerful and can cause us much joy or suffering. Without understanding how our own mind works, it is hard to know what we deeply want, where we are going in life or how we are getting there. Rather than our mind obeying *us*, we tend to obey *it*.

There is a Zen Buddhist story that illustrates this well. A man is standing beside a country road. Over the hill comes another man, on a frantically galloping horse. As horse and rider pound past in a cloud of dust, the startled onlooker shouts up to the rider, 'Wherever are you going?' The rider shakes his head helplessly, shouting back as he disappears over the next horizon, 'I don't know – ask the horse!'

Until we turn in and become acquainted with the way our own mind works, we are just like the helpless rider on the galloping horse. We remain unaware of the unconscious forces driving many of our actions. A poignant example of this occurred when I was a student. A senior professor of psychiatry was prosecuted for having shoplifted two shirts from a clothing shop. Newspapers had a field day reporting that a learned Edinburgh professor had said in court, 'I don't know why I did it.' I remember the unfairness and cruelty at the time, students and staff alike laughing as they read this. But we no more knew our own minds than the professor knew his.

At a recent exhibition at the Wellcome Trust in London[2] there was a recording of a Tibetan monk commenting on the difference between Tibetan and Western cultures. He said that he had noticed how in the West we take very good care of our bodies, how we take regular showers, perhaps even twice daily. We keep our bodies clean. In comparison, he said that many Tibetans might take a shower only once every few months, that their bodies are not as clean as ours, but added, 'We do take good care of our minds. We keep our minds clean.' He meant regular mindfulness and meditation practice.

A Few Brief Exercises (one minute each)

Just this moment, just for a moment: stop. Find a pen and a blank piece of paper to have beside you.

Now sit back comfortably in your chair – and stop again. Glance at your watch and say to yourself, 'For just a short moment, I am going to allow my mind to rest. I am going to think of absolutely nothing for the next minute.' Make that firm intention and then just do it: relax and rest in your chair, physically and mentally, for just one minute.

Did you? Did your mind rest? Or did it go on thinking? I just did this exercise too. Although I sat and firmly set the intention to rest, my mind went on thinking. My thoughts were:

- That kitchen clock has a really loud tick.
- I wonder whether I'll just irritate readers by asking them to do this.
- Must remember to buy something for supper.
- The battery on my laptop is low …Where's the lead for it?
- My left shoulder aches.

I planned to rest, but instead random thoughts kept happening. Thinking is just what the mind does, and that's

195

fine. It's helpful to get familiar with what our mind does. We think that we control our mind, but we find that it does not rest to order. Also, do we have any idea what our mind will think of next?

Again, just stop for a minute – and this time give the mind full permission to think of whatever it wants to think about. No holds barred. Sitting quietly in this space, rest and simply watch the mind. If you can, allow a few minutes to pass doing this.

Was this second exercise a little different from the first? Were there a few gaps between the thoughts this time? Just compare the two exercises lightly. Usually when we tell the mind to rest it immediately rebels and gets busy. Yet when we allow it complete freedom, saying, 'Think as much as you want, be as busy as you wish,' our mind often goes quiet for a moment. Thoughts are a little more shy in appearing.

Third quick exercise: this time give your mind no instructions at all. This time just sit for a minute and write down the first five random thoughts that come up in your mind. No censorship. Write down the first five thoughts that come, just as I wrote down mine, above.

Now look at your list of five thoughts. Did you 'decide' to think those thoughts, or did they just happen? Now notice whether perhaps you have a strong reaction to one of those thoughts. If you did, notice whether that thought has a different flavour from the others. Did you like that thought, or dislike it? Some thoughts are random and passing, they do not disturb our internal weather much. Other thoughts are sticky and come with hooks on, they bring with them a whole host of other thoughts and feelings, and suddenly we can find ourselves lost in a train of thinking that – quite literally – seems to have a mind of its own. We become the helpless rider on the galloping horse in the story.

At the beginning of one retreat I attended, Rob Nairn, a wonderful mindfulness teacher from South Africa, asked us to sit comfortably with a straight back, gently close our eyes, then allow our mind to think whatever it wanted to think. As in the exercise above, all we had to do was simply notice our thoughts as they occurred. After a minute, he sounded the bell and asked what our experience had been.

A woman in the front row immediately exploded, 'How can I possibly allow my mind to think whatever it wants to think? My first thought, and the next five thoughts too, was that I want to kill my brother-in-law.'

Unfazed, Rob answered, 'So – what's wrong with that?' She looked shocked, clearly wondering what sort of retreat she had come to. He went on. 'It's only a thought. Are you going to act on it?'

She laughed nervously. 'No, of course I'm not.'

'So, it's just a thought. Let it be. Is it there now?'

She checked and laughed again. 'No, it's not.'

By watching what went on in her mind, she was no longer afraid of her thoughts. Instead, she was aware of them.

The Vietnamese Zen Buddhist master Thich Nhat Hanh advises us to learn the art of stopping, of ceasing to be driven by our restless emotions. He states:

When an emotion rushes through us like a storm we have no peace . . . How can we stop this state of agitation? How can we stop our fear, despair, anger and craving? We can stop by practising mindful breathing, mindful walking, mindful smiling, and deep looking in order to understand.[3]

Meditation

Meditation is simply about sitting still and getting acquainted with our own mind – *all* aspects of our own mind, not just the content (our thoughts and feelings) but also the context (the spaciousness of the mind within which the thoughts arise and dissolve). It's not about forming an opinion of our mind or writing a thesis on our interesting findings, just observing very simply how thoughts arise and subside within our mind. Just watching, noting and not turning away, just as Rumi describes in the *Guest House* poem at the beginning of this chapter. Acknowledging both our thoughts and feelings, *and* our internal reactions to them, *and* the space in which everything arises and dissolves.

We are encouraged to sit with a straight back, either cross-legged on a cushion or sitting on a chair, in a posture we can rest in comfortably for ten or twenty minutes at a time. In formal meditation practice, the body is kept still so that the mind can follow suit. Body coming to rest on the cushion, mind coming to rest in the body. Body and mind together right here, right now. The intention is not to stop thoughts, rather to let them be and to simply *be aware* of the space within which they arise, show themselves, and then pass. The analogy given is that of the clear, open blue sky (the spacious *context* of the mind) and the passing moving clouds (the *content* of the mind – our thoughts and feelings). The idea is to see it all, and to rest more and more in the awareness, *as the awareness*, that sees all this.

My first meditation teacher taught us to watch our thoughts as gently and as silently as a naturalist observes nature. The image he gave was that of a watcher in a hide near a watering hole, a watcher who had an equal interest in all the animals that came to drink. Our thoughts, he said, are like those animals – they appear, stay a while at the watering hole, and then wander off again. We are the silent watcher who in no way interferes, simply observes. To judge a thought is to interfere with it; then the thought cannot fully show itself. Practising like this, we gradually drop our habitual self-judgements – not in order to be nice to ourselves; we drop the judging simply in order to be able to see what is there. For clear 360-degree seeing, only the lens of kindness will do. As we continue to meditate we may notice that we are now 'judging our judging': criticising ourselves for still having critical thoughts. No need. We allow all thoughts, generous or mean, critical or complementary, simply to be. No need to police the *content* (the thoughts that arise – they are all okay); instead we gently rest as the *context* (the awareness of all that arises).

My teacher told us not to ignore the small animals (ie the minor thoughts) that showed up, not to be overly impressed by the big ones, not to be frightened by the fierce ones, not to be fascinated by the brightly coloured ones, and not to airbrush out the dull ones. Once we start to realise that thoughts are, well, just thoughts, we can tolerate them, look at them, and so become fully aware of them. We see their nature, we see that they are indeed like clouds that arise, coalesce, then disappear within the clear, open spaciousness of the mind. No one else can see this for us.

Many thoughts pass through my mind. Of themselves they are neutral; they come and then they go. But a thought that I believe – now that's a different matter. I will act on that thought. Yet, when examined, many of the thoughts I sincerely believe about what happens to me in life turn out to be untrue. This is well illustrated by the story of a man in a boat, crossing a river in a dense mist. He paddles with great care, looking out for other boats, trying to get across the dangerous river safely. Suddenly his boat is struck by a much larger boat careering downstream. The impact nearly capsizes him. He is furious that anyone should navigate so carelessly. He stands up enraged, ready to shout abuse and fight the idiot captain of the other boat. But on standing, he sees that there is no one in the other boat.

In a sense, until each one of us turns our gaze inwards and becomes better acquainted with the way our own mind makes assumptions and then reacts, we are both the enraged man in the boat *and* the unmanned boat careering downstream. We are not awake and aware; we are not alertly helming the boat of our own mind, yet we readily vent our fury on other similarly unmanned boats around us.

Quietening down and humbly getting to know the ways of our own mind is probably the single most useful action we can take in order to lessen not just our own suffering, but the suffering of all those we impact throughout life. Buddhist teacher Yongey Mingyur Rinpoche invites us to take an honest look at ourselves and ask ourselves afresh:

What Tools Do We Need to Effect These Changes?

What do I really want out of life? Am I content to just keep improvising day to day? Am I going to ignore the vague sense of discontent that I always feel deep down when, at the same time, I am longing for well-being and fulfilment? [4]

These are certainly the questions that came into sharp focus for me when I developed cancer. If time was short, what was it that really mattered to me? None of us knows when we will die, so these are relevant questions for any of us at any time in our lives. In 2010, with a cancer recurrence, I was feeling more than 'a vague sense of discontent'. I was suffering and, in finding my life situation so difficult, I was causing suffering to others. I went for help from people who seemed to know what they were talking about, because they were calm and serene, often despite great personal suffering in the past. The unfailing instruction from all the teachers was to get to know our own mind so that we then suffer less. This was what they had done, and they were evidence of the practice. No religious allegiance required, just the simple practice of observing our own mind. I decided to give meditation and mindfulness a go.

Mindfulness

The scientist and mindfulness expert Jon Kabat-Zinn defines mindfulness as 'the awareness that emerges through paying attention on purpose, in the present moment, non-judgementally to the unfolding of experience moment by moment'. [5]

Mindfulness can therefore be practised in any posture, in any activity, at any time. We can practise mindfulness however busy our day may be – whenever that is, we remember to be mindful. Only when we are fully aware of what is happening, when it is happening (in the outer situation and also in ourselves) do we have the full information necessary to assess each situation and respond in the best way. Until I went on mindfulness courses and started to 'pay attention on purpose' to the present moment, I was genuinely unaware of how ... *unaware* I often was.

It reminded me of the feeling I get when driving with a friend of mine who has done an advanced driving course. When I drive with him I am struck by how alert his attention is when driving, how he spots the car at the junction ahead that may pull out or the motorbike behind that is about to overtake; notices slurry on the road and goes slower, anticipating the possible farm vehicle round the next bend. He didn't drive as well as this before, but he has learned to use his senses more keenly and it has now become his habit. Paying what seems like 'extra' attention does not tire him out; rather, it empowers him. While being more alert he also seems more relaxed. He is practising mindfulness while driving. Learning to make mindfulness our habit in each moment can make us all more aware, and more relaxed too.

Some people are uneasy about the recommendation in mindfulness to be *non-judgmental*. They misinterpret it as meaning, 'Become bland. Don't judge anything at all in everyday life.' Of course we have to make moment-by-moment judgments throughout each and every day in order to function. We must continue doing that. Mindfulness is simply also noticing what the processes are in our own mind as we move through our day. Only then do we come to see just how habitual most of our decisions have been, how automatic our reactions often are. It is true that regular practise of mindfulness does take the beef out of a lot of our angry agendas, and some people don't want that. What are we, after all, if we stop reacting with anger to that which offends us? Who would we be if we started to loosen our grip on our own fiercely held opinions? Wouldn't all the spice go out of our lives? The Buddhist monk Matthieu Ricard describes how we all experience and recognise 'the suffering that accompanies anger, greed or jealousy, and we all appreciate the good feelings that go along with kindness, contentment and the pleasure of seeing other people happy. The sense of harmony that is connected with loving others has an inherent goodness in it that speaks for itself.' He goes on to say that by cultivating altruistic love and inner calm our lives in fact become much richer, not less. [6]

So, given how useful mindfulness and meditation can be, how do we go about learning these new skills? Just like any new skill: we go on a course with a recognised teacher, work out whether or not this line of inquiry and practise is right for us, and if it is, commit to practising the new habits until they themselves become … habitual. This takes time. It also takes humility. We think we know all about our minds already, because each of us has a mind and because that mind has always been with us. So we believe that mindfulness will come naturally to us and will not require any marked effort on our part. When we find we cannot practise mindfulness or meditation so easily, we are often disheartened and may give up all practise, deciding this is not for us. But everyone finds it difficult to learn the new a new skill; we mustn't expect too much of ourselves in too short a time. We need to go patiently, and persistently.

Learning a new skill

I had never skied before in my life. I thought I would be a natural. As a child I used to get home from school, change my clothes, put on my roller-skates and zoom over undulating pavements to my friend Stella's house to play. She would put on her own pair and we were off, to zip around prams and elderly couples on the nearby esplanade. I used to look at grown-ups with pity. Why did they plod everywhere when they could put wheels under their feet and flow fast to every destination?

I found out why when John and I joined our children on a school skiing trip to France. At forty-two, I discovered my body was disappointingly different from that of my early years. It seemed to have forgotten all its childhood ease. Balancing on the move had fallen out of its repertoire. Why did skis have to be so *long*? Why is snow quite so *slippery*, and why do mountainsides *slope* that much? I felt incredibly unsafe. Every pine tree looked like an accident waiting to happen. The patient ski instructor told me to lean forward on my skis. I thought he must be mad. Up on the slope, as soon as I felt my skis sliding forwards under me, my instinctive reaction was to lean back, away from this dangerously accelerating downward momentum. Every time I leaned backwards, my skis and feet carried on ahead and my bruised body landed again and again on the icy snow. The ski instructor seemed to have seen this before. He just smiled patiently and kept telling me to lean forwards, to lean right into that onward movement, as only then will you stay with your skis. Only then will you have the balance to stay upright, and the power to direct your skis.

What Tools Do We Need to Effect These Changes?

Embarrassment is a powerful teacher. Our young children had also never skied before but within a morning they were whizzing happily down the slope past their parents, trying to pretend they weren't related to us. So I decided to give the crazy instructions a try. I leaned tentatively forwards and discovered to my amazement that when I did so, while I stayed wobbly, I was at least upright. I began to feel the way my skis bit into the snow whenever I leaned slightly forwards, the way they lost their purchase and slipped away from me when I leaned back. Then the instructor told me to put all my weight on one ski in order to make a turn. I discovered with delight that falling over was *not* the only way to change direction on a ski slope. This was a breakthrough. Once I also got the hang of turning my skis inwards into a snowplough I could make an ungainly descent down the mountainside, secure in the knowledge that I could at least slow down before colliding with those waiting fir trees.

It was all to do with where you put your weight, and the instructions were completely counterintuitive. My habitual reaction (to lean away from the danger) did not serve me, and I had to learn a new habit – to lean in towards the danger. To my amazement, when put into practice, this worked. If I had simply read a book about it, while never actually putting theory into practice, I would have learned nothing – no matter how animatedly I might discuss the topic with friends. I had to go to a ski slope, don a pair of skis, fall over and find out for myself whether the instructions worked or not. And they did. As a result, my confidence and trust, both in the instructions and in myself, grew. What previously had been terrifying to me became exhilarating. Once I had experienced the advice working for me even briefly, I was eager to learn more, and did not mind how many falls (and there were many) I had along the way.

Learning meditation is very similar. It is simply another new skill to learn. Strange, that most of us expect meditating to come to us easily. Hey, what's so difficult about sitting on a cushion and watching our thoughts for ten minutes? Well, just give it a go and see. I was dismayed to discover that although I had firmly set my attention to watch something as simple as my own in-breath and out-breath, my mind wandered from the task within a nanosecond. I couldn't stop thinking about what was for lunch. I nearly gave up then and there. Yet we can no more excel in our first attempts at learning to focus our attention in meditation than we can ski with grace when first pushing off on a snow-covered slope.

As with all new skills, we simply need to practise and persist. Others have learned and so can we. We take continual tumbles and accept that as part of the learning. After all, it is the only way we learned to walk in our first years of life. Learning to balance through losing balance is a well tried-and-tested method. Toddlers new on their feet don't mind the tumbles one bit. They are almost picking themselves up again before they've landed. They seem to know that we learn to walk through falling over. When do we lose this generous way of learning? Maybe when we start to take ourselves too seriously. Maybe then, our bodies and brains become more rigid, less amenable to 'learning through failing'. The good news is that both body and brain can become flexible again – if we allow them to. A sense of humour helps.

What Tools Do We Need to Effect These Changes?

Leaning into the sharp bits

The general advice given in meditation and mindfulness is similar to what I was told when learning to ski. Chögyam Trungpa advises us to: 'to lean into the sharp bits' in life. That certainly wasn't the direction I was used to leaning. Just as it had been on the ski slope, my instinct in life was to lean as far away as possible from the sharp bits. To choose to 'lean into' the sharp bits sounded plain masochistic to me. But when I did it, when I actually put it into practice, I found that everything eased. Whenever I hid from the grimness of my prognosis, turned away from the horror of maybe having only a few months or years left to live, I remained frightened and distracted, not fully present. I was overly bright in conversation and quickly tired. However, once I 'leaned into' my situation, allowed it to be just the way things were, dropping all argument and avoidance, I found to my surprise that I relaxed. I found I was far less wobbly and much less alarmed. Letting in the bad news without resistance meant I could also let in the good news without resistance. I could be fully present to enjoy the good meal, my happy family, the lovely day, the precious visiting friend.

The good news is that even for someone as lazy as me, as long as you continue to meditate for even a short time regularly, changes start to happen. Like drops of water collecting over time in a basin, nothing goes to waste. But we have to actually do it for ourselves. No one else can do it for us. A Tibetan master at Samye Ling monastery was due to give a teaching called 'Pacifying the wild mind'. However, he began by giving a teaching he called, 'Pacifying the wild belly'. He said that recently he had noticed with dismay that he was getting rather fat. He did not want to be fat, he would rather be slim; he said that he wanted to 'pacify this wild belly' of his. He thought that maybe he might need some help or advice in order to achieve his aim. So he turned to a slim member of the audience and said, 'You are not fat. You look like someone who could give me some good advice on how to lose weight. Please tell me how I can be slim too.' Then he added with great firmness, 'But first I must make a few things absolutely clear. I do not want to change what I eat. I am not prepared to eat less, and I certainly will not eat any of those so-called "health foods". Also, I have no intention of taking any exercise. Now tell me, please, I *really* want to know: how do I pacify my wild belly?'

That story will be familiar to all GPs, dieticians, health advisers and sports coaches. We desire a certain change in our bodies but would much prefer that it did not involve any commitment or – heaven forfend – discipline on our part in order to achieve it. That was the way I felt about meditation. I was interested – sure, it seemed like a good idea; yup, I'd heard there was good evidence for it working ... but this evening? I felt like relaxing and watching a film. Maybe tomorrow I'd meditate ...

I remember a Buddhist teacher talking about the Nike slogan 'Just do it.' He said, 'I don't think that slogan came about by accident. I think many sports professionals met and shared their frustration that while many customers buy all the gear, few actually run the run, cycle the bike, ever become fit. That's how those professionals got together and came up with just three practical words: 'Just *do* it.'

But before we can 'just do' mindfulness or meditation, before we can start to become acquainted with how our own mind works, we need to learn another skill that's often equally new to us – the skill of being unconditionally kind towards ourselves.

Open-eyed open-heartedness

Without kindness in our gaze, we cannot bear to look. Without calmness and non-judging we cannot bear to continue to look. Without looking we cannot understand the nature of our own mind.

> *My religion is kindness.*
>
> The Dalai Lama

If we wish to begin to observe our own mind, kindness is the only attitude that bears fruit. A harsh judging attitude only excites resistance. High expectations of ourselves have to be set aside. Gentle perseverance without expectation is the only way. Setting up impossible goals with fixed deadlines is counterproductive. Criticising ourselves for 'not having calmed the mind yet' is more of the same. Relaxing, letting be and just watching our thoughts – whatever they are, however jumbled, mean or petty they may be, in meditation, and in everyday life – is the way, and is not laxness.

> *Simply let experience take place very freely, so that your open heart is suffused with the tenderness of true compassion.*[7]
>
> Tsoknyi Rinpoche

It is remarkable to see the way people gradually change over time as their meditation practice deepens. YouTube gives us a great opportunity to see both the younger person and the older being they have grown into. I recently watched two videos of the spiritual teacher Ram Dass, the 1960s

Harvard professor who went out to India and returned to write the 1971 seminal book *Be Here Now* [8]. In the 1970s video he is bright-eyed and enthusiastic, bursting with the desire to communicate, yet I found myself unmoved. The later video touched me far more deeply. He is now in his eighties. In 1997 he suffered a major stroke. He continues to teach, despite speech difficulties and paralysis of the right side of his body. On this recent video a panel of teachers including Ram Dass was being interviewed. As the interviewer was asking another member of the panel a question, Ram Dass suddenly interrupted, saying slowly and forcefully, 'Ho … rr … i … ble thoughts, h … orr … ible thoughts.' The interviewer, clearly rather taken aback, said to him, 'But surely not right now?' and Ram Dass answered, 'Yes. R … ight … now. Horr … ible … thoughts … right … now.' There's a long pause as a slow, radiant smile spreads across his face. He beams with joy and says: 'I'll just have to … love them … to … death.' [9]

This honesty and open-hearted kindness towards yourself, towards others, even towards your own horrible thoughts, is the fruit of meditation and mindfulness practice. Whatever happens is allowed, is easily admitted. All is greeted and made welcome. Horrible thoughts do not cease to occur. But our relationship to them is utterly altered. All can be met when we have learned to relate from a place of love and acceptance.

Regret instead of guilt, forgiveness instead of condemnation

In the West, we do not readily allow, let alone love, our 'horrible thoughts'. We are much more likely to quickly judge and condemn ourselves for having them. We are so well accustomed to being self-critical and judgmental that it takes someone from outside to point this out to us. Years ago, when he first went to teach in America, the Dalai Lama was amazed to learn that self-hatred is quite common in the West. He said there was no such concept in Tibet. He found it incredible that anyone should ever hate him or herself, and listened with care and astonishment as Western students described such feelings to him.

Similarly, there is no word for 'guilt' in Tibetan. There is a word for real *regret* regarding something a person may have done – but no concept or word for that sticky, unbudging, self-condemning feeling that is *guilt*. Deeply felt regret is painful but it is also liberating; it motivates us to change our behaviour. Deeply felt *guilt* has a different tone: it immobilises and transfixes, is hard to move on from.

Guilt never features in Tibetan stories. Instead there are riveting tales of persons who have committed a multitude of fairly horrendous actions such as killing and stealing yet who nonetheless succeed in reaching enlightenment after meeting the teachings of the Buddha, deeply regretting their past behaviour, and radically altering their lives in line with those teachings. Changes then happen, even to them. No one, but no one, is excluded from this possibility of changing.

Present-day research in neuroscience confirms that our brain – everyone's brain – is capable of change both in behaviour and structure over time. Yongey Mingyur Rinpoche states that during his discussions with scientists across the globe he has been struck by the 'nearly universal consensus in the scientific community that the brain is structured in a way that actually does make it possible to effect real changes in everyday experience'. [10]

Six

Many Paths, Same Destination

The teachers of mindfulness, meditation, Buddhism, Christian mysticism, Sufiism, Advaita Vedanta and others all seem to have a similar underlying message: to be more aware, more present in the moment (which is all that we ever have); to be kinder, more forgiving, more tolerant human beings; to come to realise that we are much vaster and much more interconnected with each other and everything in the universe than we take ourselves to be.

They all speak of the same themes and give similar advice:

1. Investigate what is your view – of life, of
    yourself – because that will determine your
    actions, and your actions in this moment
    determine your future.
2. Practise …
    Kindness
    Tolerance and acceptance
    Humility and humour
    Compassion and forgiveness of self and other

Appreciation, gratitude and generosity
Patience and perseverance in developing these qualities

3. Recognise how everything in ourselves and in the world is impermanent (constantly changing) and interdependent (dynamically interrelating). Enjoy the vastness and beauty of that.

I was struck by the deep, underlying similarities in all the teachings I had explored. When I spoke with Lama Yeshe about this he briskly said, 'Yes, yes. All teachers of truth are saying the same thing.' My stunning insight didn't amaze him in the slightest. A little worried that I was shopping around the spiritual marketplace excessively, I went on to say that in writing this book about all the help he had given me, I would also want to write of the help my mother's Catholic priest had given me. Lama Yeshe responded enthusiastically. 'Good, good. Write the book and tell them you have *double* pedigree.'

I burst out laughing and said I was more of a happy mongrel. My Anglican Catholic mother and my Scottish Presbyterian father would have approved.

Brother David's teaching

Brother David Steindl-Rast grew up in Austria during the Second World War. He described boys older than him completing school only to soon die as soldiers. He fully expected to follow them, but then the war ended and suddenly he was a carefree university student. He became a Benedictine monk aged twenty-nine and is now over ninety. He teaches with a sparkle and gratitude for life that is infectious. He says he doesn't use the word 'God' as people have so many different ideas of what God is. Instead he talks of that which we all have to relate to – life.

He asks, 'What is life?' He describes how you cannot grasp life; rather, that life grasps you (just as we cannot 'grasp' music; instead it grasps us). Life is mystery, but it is not mystifying. He describes hope as 'the openness to surprise' and recommends that we wake each day with gratitude, and say to life, 'Surprise me!' When we live like that, with trust in life, our doing will be love. He describes love as 'a wholehearted "Yes!" to mutual belonging'. Only then can we understand life, because only then are we present. When we enter fully into life we continually encounter mystery. Then we are 'present' – 'when heart speaks to heart'. We are present to everything – other people, animals, plants, the earth itself.

When we ask ourselves, 'Who is present?' each one of us answers 'I, I myself.' He asks each of us to watch our self, to become the watcher. He asks, 'Is that watcher also being watched?' and adds, 'When you are the watcher that no one can watch, then you are the self. The self is not in time and space; rather, it observes time and space. There is only one self and we all share it.' He describes how we are each unique as an individual 'I' in time and space, but that we all also share this one universal self that is outside of time and space. The one self is playing all the roles. So the 'I myself' is in fact the universal timeless self as well as the unique individual 'I' in time and space. [1]

This matches exactly the Buddhist teachings on relative and ultimate reality. We exist in the world as an individual person, an 'I', but at the same time our true nature is the universal self that is timeless, spaceless, traceless.

The analogy given by the Vietnamese Zen Buddhist master Thich Nhat Hanh is that of a wave on the ocean. A wave exists in time and space, comes into being and then breaks on the shore. If the wave sees its identity only as 'I am wave' then it will be intimidated by other waves, mourn its own short life and feel very insecure in the middle of the vast ocean. However if the wave recognises its true nature, 'I am water', it realises that it is indestructible, that there is nothing to fear – it is one with the whole ocean. It sees that ceasing to be a wave makes no difference. Even if it evaporates from the ocean surface it will become a cloud, fall as rain, return to the ocean in a river. There is nothing it can fear once it recognises itself both as 'wave' and as 'water'. [2]

Brother David describes how, when we know that we are both the universal self and the individual I, we can play our individual role well and live with joy and trust. However, when the individual 'I' forgets that its true nature is universal self, it becomes fearful and shrivels down into a frightened ego that believes it is separate from all that is. Like a wave that forgets that its true nature is water, the frightened ego forgets that it is interrelated with all that is. It believes itself to be alone. In its fright it then grabs hold of people, money, status – anything for security (grasping); and then has to defend these precious possessions from all comers (aggression). And the more we accrue, the more we have to defend, and the deeper our sense of loneliness and isolation becomes.

My understanding of the teachings

When trouble hits, when our world is shaken for whatever reason, we tend initially to grab on to what we already know. But often this set of beliefs from yesterday cannot serve us well, as we are now meeting a larger reality that requires a wider vision and different, fresh responses. That's when we need help in finding a greater spaciousness to experience all this in. When my cancer recurred I was terrified and I needed help. I went to many different teachers, attended a variety of retreats. The sceptic in me questioned whether I wasn't just seeking straws to grab hold of. Instead I found bedrock to stand on, and I found it everywhere.

The message running through all the teachings I found can be summed up in seven points:

1. You are not who or what you think you are; you are not who or what you take yourself to be. You are much, much more than that.

2. Find out who you truly are. Enquire within. This is possible.

3. Move helpfully in the world, recognising that all beings want to be happy just as you do, but accept that the only part of the world you have the power to change is … you.

4. Everything in our internal and external world is interdependent with everything else, so when you change internally, everything changes externally. This is the power you do have.

5. Do not try to forcibly rearrange reality to better meet your needs. This is the power you don't have. You are free to try, but you'll lose every time. If you keep at it, your life becomes a life of aggression, fighting and constant complaint. This is wearisome for you, your family and the world. It is also futile.

6. Drop the victim mentality. We are mainly our own victims. If we believe we are powerless, well then – we are. Start trusting life. Start trusting yourself. Experiment and find out for yourself. You are your own authority.
7. Open your heart. Lean into the sharp bits. Let go of fear and grow in love.

This wasn't really what I'd been looking for. It all sounded a bit much. This required a fundamental shift in how I looked at life and called for more hard work, internally, than I felt ready for. This would take courage. I was tired physically and emotionally, and my courage stores felt pretty depleted. As far as I was concerned, I'd already leaned into more than enough sharp bits in recent years. I felt protective of myself and did not initially warm to such teachings. I can remember even finding them unkind.

I kept moving on, looking for wisdom in an easier form. I didn't find it. Instead I kept meeting the same message in a different guise. I tried returning to my 'old way of seeing' but that didn't work either; it no longer satisfied. If anything, I felt a bit homeless. So despite feeling almost repelled by the bluntness of the message I found, I kept returning to read the books that said these odd things about compassion being the strongest force in the universe; attending talks from teachers who spoke with ease from a place I didn't quite get; I kept hanging back yet moving closer – 'circling the drain' as Adyashanti puts it. Something strongly attracted me to the core of these teachings but I was wary. I sensed that everything I had previously taken for granted would be thrown into question, so I approached slowly. I wanted – but I also didn't want – deep change.

My investigation of these different ways of seeing was persistent but somewhat meandering, and pretty slow. Given that I had, and still have, an incurable cancer, it may seem odd that despite sensing their truth, I took my time. But deep attraction also excites an equal and opposite resistance. I was deeply reluctant to let go of any part of my existing way of seeing. It had got me this far, given me a certain security, protected me in part. If I let go of that – what then? I wasn't ready to trade my view for a vaster view. It felt too risky, even agoraphobic, when these teachers talked of a love so vast that hatred and fear – of anything under the sun – simply ceases to be a possibility. They then went on to say that this vastness of love was our basic nature, our fundamental truth; that this unconditional love is who we really are. Heck, who would I be if I went along with *that?* Sounded to me like far too many of my defences would have to be thrown to the wind, and I was feeling vulnerable enough already.

But then I looked at Lama Yeshe and Akong Rinpoche. I looked at Thich Nhat Hanh. I saw Father MacLean's and Brother David Steindl-Rast's glow and enthusiasm for life – all of life. I watched the way the Dalai Lama walks on to a stage, any stage, and meets the world. I watched him on YouTube giggling merrily as he shared a joke with Archbishop Desmond Tutu – these two men who must have heard some of the saddest stories of humanity and never flinched. I might find the teachings of Buddha and Christ too much at times, but neither could I move away from the people who truly embodied these teachings. They had such a remarkable way of being human. They were so clearly there for others, having no demands for themselves. They fully allowed in all the pain of the world, devoted their lives to lessening it, yet carried themselves lightly.

Putting this into everyday practice: The Middle Way
One summer I went on a retreat at Plum Village, the Buddhist community founded by Thich Nhat Hanh, who is also known as 'Thay', or teacher. Thay grew up in a Vietnam on fire, his country occupied by American soldiers fighting the Viet Cong. Disappointed with the response of the Buddhist religious establishment to the suffering of the villagers, Thay founded a movement of young monastics who went into the bombed-out, napalmed villages to help the peasants rebuild their homes and replant their crops.

The young monks and nuns refused to take sides with either warring party. They simply worked for peace in the midst of war. As a result they were in grave danger from both sides: the Viet Cong suspected them of being CIA agents, the Americans suspected them of being Viet Cong. Some of their number were shot and killed. Still they went and helped the people, among them Sister Chan Khong. This young Vietnamese woman went up-river, cross-country and into the most dangerous urban areas of Vietnam, taking food and medicines to those in need during the war. She was tireless, and even when exiled with Thay to France, she set up a system whereby donors in the West could help orphaned children in Vietnam.

Sister Chan Khong now lives and teaches at Plum Village, looking after nuns and retreatants from almost every country in the world. She is a legend in her own right, a human dynamo of compassionate activity. I felt very lucky on my retreat that visitors were able to have an interview with her. She was so easy to talk with, and such a good listener, that I found myself describing to her my life as a rural doctor, a wife, a mother and daughter.

At the time, my mother was still alive, widowed and very unhappy in nearby sheltered housing, and she wanted me to visit her frequently. I was in the typical position of a busy working mum, needing to care for the generation above as our parents got frailer, needing to care for the generation below as our children turned into teenagers. You relate to your spouse mainly by saying, 'Could you pick up some milk/bread/one of our children on your way back from ...' Mum was unhappy on her own and I always went when she asked, while worrying that I was short-changing John and the children. It was the same when I worked late at the surgery, seeing extra patients. I felt pulled in all directions. All I knew was that I was doing nothing well.

Sister Chan Khong smiled and said, 'So, you are not queen of your own kingdom.'

Kingdom? No one had ever told me I had one of those. I was confused by the question, coming from someone who did so much more for others than I ever could.

I parried: 'But surely you do so much more than me, you meet all the requests for help that come to you? You are always giving of yourself.'

'Yes, but it is I who decides what I do. I am always queen of my own kingdom. If someone comes into your kingdom with loud insistent demands, you must politely ask them to sit down, to quieten down a little. This is your kingdom, and you are queen here. A kingdom has boundaries and also has guards at the gates who are permitted to ask people – even mothers – to wait a little before entering too forcefully.'

Well! This was news to me – news I put into firm action once I got home. And of course, Sister Chan Khong's advice echoed Thay's own teaching. At Plum Village, the community have a weekly 'lazy day' when the monks and nuns rest, go for walks, maybe have a picnic, make no demands on themselves ... other than to do nothing. Meetings that have not been fitted into their otherwise busy week are not allowed to fill this day. Some of the Western monastics did not like the term 'lazy day' and wanted to rename it 'rest day' but Thay insisted: this was a day to relax and practise *laziness*. If we do not relax we cannot nourish ourselves. True tolerance and compassion also means saying a clear 'No' when the demand is excessive, and taking a rest. You are reminded to include yourself in the field of compassion: no one gets left out of this love, not even you. The advice is to keep everything in balance, not to pursue extremes, rather to find the middle way between those extremes; to find a way for our self that is both possible and authentic.

Even our own heart, that faithful muscle which pumps blood around our body day and night, has a contraction phase and a relaxation phase within each heartbeat, relaxation being as vital as contraction. If the heart muscle does not fully relax and dilate, the chambers inside it do not fill up with sufficient blood. This means that when the heart muscle then contracts, insufficient blood is pumped into the arterial systems of the body. Heart efficiency is a factor both of heart contractility and heart relaxability.

Thay sees that we have in part forgotten how to relax, that

we need to relearn and practise a better balance between working and resting. He teaches compassion, nothing but compassion, but also advises us against taking on more than we have the present capacity for:

> *If we feel there is someone we cannot help, it is only because we have not yet looked deeply enough into his or her circumstances.*

> *If we open our hearts freely, but do not know our own limitations, our own seeds of agitation will be watered and we will become overwhelmed.* [3]
>
> *Thich Nhat Hanh*

On the last day of the retreat, Thay said he hoped that each participant would go home feeling more deeply rooted both in their own culture and in their own religion. He required no one to become anything else; he wished only for us to become more fully and joyfully what we already were.

Living with uncertainty

The possibility of being aware, of gathering information while not instantly calling in the jury; of discerning what is going on with an open mind; of mulling over differing possibilities; of allowing for the fact that there is usually so much that we do *not* know: this is the highest scientific discipline, and the method and foundation of all scientific discovery.

> *I think that when we know that we actually do live in uncertainty, then we ought to admit it; it is of great value*

to realise that we do not know the answers to different questions. This attitude of mind – this attitude of uncertainty – is vital to the scientist, and it is this attitude of mind which the student must first acquire. [4]

Richard Feynman

We agree that an open mind is vital for understanding a scientific problem. Unless we allow in all the evidence impartially, how can we come to a valid conclusion? Yet we only have to glance at our newspapers and TV screens to know that this is not how we form our view about the world in general. Dramatic disaster headlines sell papers, as do outrageous statements by politicians seeking publicity – our eye is drawn to them. Twenty-four-hour news channels gather more regular listeners if they begin and end with items that heighten our anxiety – our ear is then drawn to tune in again and listen to the next news bulletin. We have been made anxious so we need to hear more, in order to reassure ourselves. It is simple marketing and social manipulation. It works both for the media moguls whose profits soar and for the global or national powers pulling the strings.

It works less well for society. Increased fear makes us less trusting, less open to each other. When frightened, we reach more rapidly for simplistic solutions. Our minds close. We become quick to judge, solidify and condemn. The nasty hunt for a scapegoat can begin. When fear is rife, facts get pushed to one side. Manipulators of power know this and use it to their advantage. Confusion soars and it can become difficult to find a way back. This is where the simple but profound practice of meditation and mindfulness can help us find much-needed space. Opening ourselves to wider possibilities, to wider ways of looking, can help centre us again and give us a calm space in which to assess what is going on.

Who do we take ourselves, the ones experiencing this life, to be?

> *The first principle is that you must not fool yourself, and*
> *you are the easiest person to fool.* [5]
>
> *Richard Feynman*

The biggest assumption we ever make in life is that we are a separate entity – separate from each other and separate from the world. Me over here, you over there. This assumption makes us more lonely than every other assumption put together. Of course it *seems* that each person is a separate entity functioning fairly autonomously, but if we rationally and logically investigate both ourselves and others it is very hard to find the actual boundary where 'other' stops and 'I' begins ...

Investigating our idea of our separate identity in terms of time:

In genetic terms every cell of our body is made up – literally formed by – the DNA of our mother and the DNA of our father, their cells in turn were formed by the DNA of their parents, their parents' cells by their parents' ... and so on and so on, back to the beginning of human history and before. So it is accurate to say that we are not only continuous with, but are actually made of, everything that has gone before. The past is not only in us, it *is* us. Then the anthropologists inform us that all human beings are originally descended from only seven women. That puts a spanner in our notions of firm and fixed ethnic divisions across the globe: we are more interlinked than we assumed. All historic events that have ever occurred form the shape of the world we live in now, and this present moment is the ground for all the events that will ever occur in the future.

Even the concept of the 'present moment' does not stand up to close examination. We use the term for 'this moment right now' – the moment that exists between past (what has been) and future (what is yet to come). So the present moment rests on a knife edge between a past that has just this moment ceased to happen and a future that has not yet occurred. How long is the duration of this 'present moment'? Does the 'now' last a second, a nanosecond, a tiny fraction of a nanosecond, or is it shorter still? But in the present moment the past is not here – it has already gone; the future is not here either – it has yet to appear. So 'past' and 'future' actually only exist as concepts, highly useful concepts, in our heads … in the present moment. So the 'now' is all we ever have at any point in time, the past being simply our memory, the future being merely our imagination.

And then the quantum physicists come along and tell us that their experiments have discovered sub-atomic particles that behave as if they are moving backwards in time; and even more unnervingly that two entangled particles (particles formed in the same event) will always demonstrate what Einstein coined 'spooky action at a distance', when two entangled particles undergo corresponding changes at exactly the same time, even if they are separated by millions of miles of space.

Maybe time and space are much more fluid than we have generally assumed them to be – as we also are, in the midst of shifting space and time.

Investigating our idea of separate identity in terms of space:

We have seen how we are not separate from our forebears in time, but are we also as separate from each other in space as we assume? Where precisely do I end and you begin? When we sit in a crowded room together we are literally breathing in and out air that only moments earlier was the breath of our neighbour. If you say something that deeply upsets me, your words remain in my head, forming a part of who I now am, affecting my responses maybe for years to come. If you sing a song I find sweet, or read a moving poem to me, then that product of your activity becomes a part of me too. If someone loves us when we are young and vulnerable, that love stays within us, giving us confidence throughout life. It is an integral part of who we are. We are social beings who affect each other and interact with each other deeply. We are made of each other.

Humanly, but also functionally, we are all interconnected. I am typing this in my kitchen on a computer made in China, sitting on a chair that comes from IKEA, my feet resting on old kitchen slabs that must have been carted here from a quarry in Scotland, wrapped in a shawl made in India (it's a Scottish kitchen after all), drinking a beer made in Prague, looking through spectacle frames made in Denmark. If I reflect on how many actual people across the world I need to extend my thanks to for my comfortable evening as I write this, the list is overwhelming.

Earlier today I was in an Edinburgh supermarket ordering some photo prints. I was struggling with the technology as I chose which images I wanted from my camera card. The person behind the counter helped me so tactfully and courteously that we got talking. He said he was glad simply to have a job. I couldn't place his accent. As I left, I asked him where he was from (just what my mother used to do, to my mortification, and now here I am doing the same). He explained that his mother was Scottish, his father Iranian, and then blurted out that his father had died only a few months ago in Iran and that he had never been able to go back to see his father in the past twenty years, not even when he was ill. Shocked, I asked why not. He answered, 'I once served in the British army. The authorities would think me a spy and imprison me.' The poignancy of a son unable to get back to his father ... He is in my mind, too, as I type this. Now he is in this book, and in your mind too as you in turn read these words. We are all made up of each and every interaction we have with each other.

Thich Nhat Hanh writes, 'There is a cloud floating in this paper.' He explains to the reader of his book that without a cloud forming in the sky, rain falling, a tree growing, a lumberjack cutting it down, the lumberjack's parents giving birth to the lumberjack, the paper mill pulping the wood to make paper, the people who work in that mill ... there would be no paper to form the book that they are now reading.

He calls this relationship 'interbeing'. And so we 'inter-are' with the plants and trees around us, too. Plants need the carbon dioxide in our outbreath as much as we need the oxygen that they put out into the atmosphere. Without plants first having the capacity to harness the energy of the sun with chorophyll, there would have been no food to sustain animals, no human evolution. As Thich Nhat Hanh teaches, we are interdependent with, not separate from, all other beings, plants, and the earth itself and we need to treat them all with equal tenderness and compassion. They are our home. [6]

The interrelatedness of scientific thought and religious thought

Since everything in the universe 'inter-is', or interweaves, with every single other thing in the universe, I include here some quotations from famous physicists, all Nobel prizewinners. They describe not only the interweaving of scientific thinking and religious thinking, but also the interweaving between 'external' object and 'internal' subject. It would seem that all such separations exist only in our heads, are just ways in which we've sought to separate and dissect the inseparable interactive world we live in.

Albert Einstein (1879–1955)

A human being is a part of a whole, called by us 'Universe', a part limited in time and space. He experiences himself, his thoughts and feelings as something separated from the rest – a kind of optical delusion of his consciousness. This delusion is a kind of prison for us, restricting us to our personal desires and to affection for a few persons nearest to us. Our task must be to free from this prison by widening our circle of compassion to embrace all living creatures and the whole nature in its beauty. [7]

Science without religion is lame. Religion without science is blind. [8]

I like to experience the universe as one harmonious whole. Every cell has life. Matter, too, has life; it is energy solidified. [9]

Richard Feynman (1918–1988)

The internal machinery of life, the chemistry of the parts, is something beautiful. And it turns out that all life is interconnected with all other life. [10]

Nature uses only the longest threads to weave her patterns, so that each small piece of her fabric reveals the organisation of the entire tapestry. [11]

Neils Bohr (1885–1962)

I myself find the division of the world into an objective and a subjective side much too arbitrary. The fact that religions through the ages have spoken in images, parables, and paradoxes means simply that there are no other ways of grasping the reality to which they refer. But that does not mean that it is not a genuine reality. And splitting this reality into an objective and a subjective side won't get us very far. [12]

A physicist is just an atom's way of looking at itself. [13]

Erwin Schrödinger (1887–1961)

The world is given to me only once, not one existing and one perceived. Subject and object are only one. The barrier

between them cannot be said to have broken down as a
result of recent experience in the physical sciences, for this
barrier does not exist. [14]

Werner Heisenberg (1901–1976)

Revere those things beyond science which really matter
and about which it is so difficult to speak. [15]

In the history of science, ever since the famous trial of
Galileo, it has repeatedly been claimed that scientific truth
cannot be reconciled with the religious interpretation of
the world. Although I am now convinced that scientific
truth is unassailable in its own field, I have never found
it possible to dismiss the content of religious thinking as
simply part of an outmoded phase in the consciousness
of mankind, a part we shall have to give up from now
on. Thus, in the course of my life I have repeatedly been
compelled to ponder on the relationship of these two
regions of thought, for I have never been able to doubt the
reality of that to which they point. [16]

★ ★ ★

My dad, a humble Scottish maths and physics teacher,
would shake with laughter to be included amongst these
august scientists, but I feel he summed up the same
message about the interconnectedness of the observed and
the observer, of the inter-being of us and our world, in
the following poem he wrote about the Cornish sea after
a fierce storm:

The Bay Looked West

Today, bright morning and the long green waves,
Late echoes of some far Atlantic quarrel;
The night-built scene lay open to the sun
In all the pomp of an advancing army.
The mile-wide ranks were faultlessly aligned,
Unhurried, confident of vast reserves,
So they came on, and as they neared the shore
The off-shore wind awarded them their plumes,
And they came faster, startlingly taller, prouder.

And it was then I knew
That who observes indeed participates;
My thought now lent the lip-curl its contempt,
Infused with dread the rearing wall of water
And crashed a challenge to the watching cliffs;
Then sped in glee across the rock-strewn beach,
Dissolving in white laughter.
Implicit, too, the sense of being observed
By waves and cliffs, all vibrantly aware,
Curious spectators, like those daffodils
That watched a poet dancing. [17]

AJ Gunn

Just as Neils Bohr could see himself, a physicist, as being just 'an atom's way of looking at itself', my dad, too, saw reciprocity and interconnectedness in everything and could enjoy musing on those Lake District daffodils that gazed back at the poet Wordsworth.

The kingdom is within
All the major world religions point towards a unity, a harmony. They point to a centre that is everywhere, and is within each one of us. They point to that centre being love.

Carved on the temple of Apollo in Delphi, Ancient Greece

Gnothi seauton – know thyself.

Luke 17: 20–21, King James Bible

When asked by the Pharisees when the kingdom of God would come, Jesus answered, 'Neither shall they say, Lo here! or, lo there! for behold, the kingdom of God is within you.'

Ancient Egyptian proverb

The kingdom of heaven is within you; and whosoever shall know himself shall find it.

Prophet Muhammad (570–632 AD)

. . . and He is with you wherever you are. [18]

My mercy embraces all things. [19]

Ibn 'Arabi (1165–1240 AD), Sufi scholar

He who knows his own self knows his Lord.

Rabbi Jonathan Sacks, Judaic scholar

Love is what redeems us from the prison cell of the self and all the sickness to which the narcissistic self is prone.

Acts of kindness can never die. They linger in the memory, giving life to other acts in return.

The only force equal to a fundamentalism of hate is a counter-fundamentalism of love. [20]

Adi Shankara, Hindu and Advaita Vedanta, philosopher (eighth century)

Curb your senses and your mind and see the Lord within your heart. [21]

Guru Nanak, founder of Sikhism (1469–1539)

As fragrance abides in the flower, as the reflection is within the mirror, so doth the Lord abide within thee. Why search Him without? [22]

Lao Tzu, founder of Taoism (604–531 BC)

Worlds and particles, bodies and beings, time and space: all are transient expressions of the Tao. [23]

Black Elk, Native American spiritual leader (1863–1950)

The Great Spirit is everywhere; He hears whatever is in our minds and hearts, and it is not necessary to speak to Him in a loud voice. [24]

The first peace ... is that which comes within the souls of men when they realise their relationship, their oneness, with the universe and all its powers ... and they realise that ... this centre is really everywhere, it is within each of us. [25]

Nisargadatta Maharaj, Indian sage (1897–1981)
> *When I look inside and see that I am nothing, that is wisdom.*
>
> *When I look outside and see that I am everything, that is love.*
>
> *And between the two, my life turns.* [26]

In my understanding, the Buddhist view is that we are not the limited person we take, or rather 'mis-take' ourselves to be. Our true nature is pure, good, loving and vast beyond our imagining. The teachings state that we fail to recognise our true nature because it is:

Too close – we are it, and therefore we cannot see it; we can only be it.

Too simple – we believe we are more difficult, more sophisticated, more complex.

Too vast – we try to fit the vastness of who and what we really are into the smallness of who we have assumed ourselves to be until now. This is not possible. However, it is possible to simply let go of our misperceived littleness, realise that we are the vastness (and have been all along), at the same time realising that everyone and everything else is also that vastness. There is no higher or lower. We can relax because we are equal and interconnected with all things.

Too good – *No, that cannot possibly be me. I'm poor, miserable and far too unworthy to be associated with, let alone 'be', unconditional love.*

Christian mystics also point to this same inner vastness, peace and purity when describing their practice of silent contemplation:

St Teresa of Avila, Carmelite abbess (1515–1582)

Everything is stilled and the soul is left in a state of great quiet and deep satisfaction . . . From this there sometimes springs an interior peace and quietude which is full of happiness. Even speaking – by which I mean vocal prayer and meditation – wearies it: it would like to do nothing but love. [27]

Thomas Merton, Trappist monk (1915–1968)

The utter simplicity and obviousness of the infused light which contemplation pours into our soul suddenly awakens us to a new level of awareness. We enter a region which we had never even suspected, and yet it is this new world which seems familiar and obvious. The old world of our senses is now the one that seems to us strange, remote, unbelievable . . . A door opens in the centre of our being and we seem to fall through it into immense depths which, although they are infinite, are all accessible to us; all eternity seems to have become ours in this one placid and breathless contact. [28]

The two movements

The teacher Adyashanti, or Adya, describes two complementary movements of spiritual awakening, the one
manifested in the life of Shakyamuni Buddha, the other
manifested in the life of Jesus Christ: [29]

Up and out

Adya describes how, in 500 BC, the Indian prince Siddhartha
left his palace and after years of intense meditative practice
woke 'up and out of' normal human consciousness into
divine consciousness, or full awareness, thus becoming the
Buddha – 'the one who is awake'. The Buddha went on
to found a monastic order and taught 'only the nature of
suffering and the cessation of suffering' for the rest of his life.

Down and in

Adya describes how, in contrast, divine consciousness
descended 'down and into' Jesus of Nazareth on his baptism
in the river Jordan, divine consciousness then becoming fully
embodied in man. This was when the man Jesus became the
awakened being Christ. Christ gathered disciples and taught,
but he did not found a monastic contemplative order. His
path was an embodied one within the world – love made
flesh and dwelling among us.

Adya describes how many spiritual seekers today want to
wake 'up and out of' the world – and then to rest there (in
serene transcendence). However, he describes that when,
through grace, anyone experiences an awakening, the call is
then to return 'down and into' the world, to fully re-engage
in order to become embodied love in service to the world;
in order to allow and be both movements of awakening.

The Indian sage Nisargadatta described how, after awakening to our true nature, our sole concern is then 'to ease the senseless sorrow of mankind'.

The thirteenth-century Islamic scholar and Sufi mystic Jalāl ad-Dīn Muhammad Rūmī wrote the following poem, which puts aside all reference points, leaving only – love:

Only Breath

Not Christian or Jew or Muslim, not Hindu,
Buddhist, Sufi, or Zen. Not any religion

or cultural system. I am not from the East
or the West, not out of the ocean or up

from the ground, not natural or ethereal, not
composed of elements at all. I do not exist,

am not an entity in this world or in the next,
did not descend from Adam and Eve or any

origin story. My place is placeless, a trace
of the traceless. Neither body or soul.

I belong to the beloved, have seen the two
worlds as one and that one call to and know,

First, last, outer, inner, only that
Breath breathing human being. [30]

(Reproduced here with the kind permission
of the translator, Coleman Barks)

Part Three

Steer Your Own Course

Love In a Time of Fear

One essential aspect of all the seminars, courses and retreats that I went to – courses on yoga, tai chi, mindfulness, Buddhism, Christian mysticism, Sufiism, Advaita Vedanta, anthroposophy, Jungian analysis (at least I was wide open in my looking, no strong prejudices against any one creed or discipline) – was that no one ever asked me to 'join up' or even suggested that I should. I would have veered away immediately if they had.

I laugh as I reread what I've just written, as right there on the page is my strong belief (verging on prejudice) that no one should ever influence another person to join their church or religion. Folk should leave other people full space to find their own way in life. So, given that belief, whatever am I doing writing a book like this: a book offering diverse ways of looking at the world, many of those ways stemming from ancient religions? Am I now doing what I've always criticised others for doing? Well, maybe I am, but I sincerely hope that I'm not. I am never once saying 'join' anything. My understanding, my underlying sense, from all these teachings is that none of us needs feel that we have to join anything – we are already complete and beautiful as we are. It is just that we do not know it.

My motivation is only to pass on to others what helped me in a practical way when I was in a tight place. And what helped me was to meet others who were calm despite a storm raging around them, who were not withdrawn but moved usefully to help those in need, who had full confidence in themselves while never taking themselves too seriously; people who seemed able to weather the worst yet also be joyful. How did they do that?

> *I find hope in the darkest of days*
> *and focus in the brightest.*
> *I do not judge the universe.*[1]
>
> *The Dalai Lama*

Once my cancer recurred and could not be cured, I asked what did I really want in life now, in this short time I had left? Very simple answers came: I wanted as much quality time as possible with my precious family and friends; I wanted to be more *alive*, more authentic; I wanted to find a way to lessen the fear that froze me; and I wanted to share what I learned along the way. When I met or saw individuals full of kindness and compassion – from whatever religion, or none – who had a certain confidence and ease, come what may, I realised I wanted to be the way they were. I, too, wanted to take life lightly, even joyfully, while backing away from nothing. So I listened to what they had to say. I was drawn to Buddhist teachings mainly because the Buddha emphasises again and again to his listeners that they should not believe anything he said but instead examine his teachings carefully, test them out, see if they are of value or not – and to go on doing this. He urges us *to find out for ourselves*, constantly discarding what we find to be false, but assimilating what we test and find to be true.

Some of what has helped me may resonate with you. Some may seem odd or even deeply jar with you. If there are any parts of this book you deeply disagree with, please just dismiss them. I am bound to have made mistakes or have been unskilful in describing the themes running through the teachings that have most helped me. Leave any parts that irritate to one side, read other, better, books on anything that may have stimulated your interest; move on. All that matters is what is true for you in *your* life. Nothing else will do.

Make your own sandwiches

I heard recently of a schoolteacher in San Francisco who became concerned by the increasing number of homeless and hungry people living on the streets in her city. She decided that if she had the energy after a day's teaching, she would make up a basket of sandwiches each afternoon and hand these around to the folk sitting in the street. No one had to be grateful. It was simply that she had food and they did not. Local radio heard about her and ran a story on what she was doing. To her surprise, she started getting donations of money in her mailbox. Donors, however, were surprised in turn when they got their money sent back to them, with a slip inside the envelope that read, *Make your own damn sandwiches*.

This story really appealed to me. In fact, that teacher has unwittingly been the stimulus for me to complete this book.

In the autumn of 2016 I was feeling particularly autumnal. I felt deeply discouraged by the state of the world today: our post-war baby boom generation was such a lucky one – couldn't we have done better than this? We could have achieved so much in terms of universal justice and feeding the hungry in the world. Instead we've had wars, famines, refugee crises, banking crises, increasing pollution, climate change and the rich getting ever richer in an economy premised on profit alone. I was wistful, too, because in the past I would have dealt with my dismay by doing something similar to this straightforward Californian woman. But my energy and health are both too variable now for me to go out and be useful in a local food bank.

Then I realised that my story about living with fear, about being helped to find new ways of responding to difficult times – that this was the sandwich I could make and offer to others. I don't know if my story is appetising or even edible to readers, but it is the only one I have to offer. The San Francisco woman's advice applies to us all: we all have unique stories and unique skills. Only we can know what it is that we have to offer to ourselves and to our world. Only we can decide what it is, that only we can give, that will help another. Only we can 'make our own damn sandwiches'. So if I had a mantra, it would be:

Steer your own course, decide for yourself . . . And make your own sandwiches!

Our power as individuals is in how we respond – and that power is limitless

Each of us meets the challenges in our lives as best we can. We cannot judge our own lives by anyone else's. Reading about the lives of Mahatma Gandhi, Nelson Mandela, Thich Nhat Hanh, Akong Rinpoche and Lama Yeshe, we may be inspired, but we may also compare our own lives and achievements with theirs and feel daunted. It is important not to go down that route. The bravest man in a village I once worked in lived alone, wrapped in a chronic state of agitated depression. He had phobias about leaving the house, touching door handles, meeting others, treading on dog dirt in the street. Everyday activity was a source of terror to him. When I saw him out doing his shopping, I knew that he had more courage than anyone else I would meet that day.

There is a similar risk in writing a book about having cancer. Others may think that their problems should no longer matter in comparison. This is not true. I think one of the hardest times in my life was when I had mild postnatal depression as a young mother. My life looked happy and fortunate to others but I was barely coping. I had every reason to be happy but it has never been harder for me to get up each morning and go through the motions of the day. I was helped enormously, as I am now, by friends who simply listened, who didn't judge, who just were there for me. When I confided in one friend how desperate I was feeling, she said, 'Mary, sometimes the bravest thing we ever do is simply put supper on the table each day.' She was right.

So above all, we need to be kind and generous to ourselves as we meet our own challenges. One teacher said, 'Do not compare your own suffering with another's. Your own suffering is more than enough for you.' And we all need to remember our own simple power to effect change in the world, just through the way we are. It is said that a kind act has a knock-on effect all around: someone who has just received kindness is kinder to the next person they interact with. We wield great power in the quality of our interactions with each other, moment by moment.

> *The present moment*
> *contains past and future.*
> *The secret of transformation*
> *is in the way we handle this very moment* [2]
>> *Thich Nhat Hanh*

The world today

We can often feel overwhelmed when we turn on the news channels and hear and see reports of the troubled world. The sheer scale of anger, misery and ongoing conflict in so many areas can make us want to turn off, to turn away. I write this the day after the 2016 American election, the end of a bruising fight for America and for all who watched what came to feel increasingly like a blood sport. The rhetoric was vitriolic and was amplified by being rapidly fed and retweeted across the internet. The president-elect is an unknown quantity, even to himself. America is deeply divided and the world is edgy. Vital international climate agreements now appear shaky. In the Middle East, the tragic aftermath of past interventions is being played out in the homes of the people of Mosul, Raqqa and Aleppo. Barrel bombs in Aleppo and mass graves in Islamic State held areas of war-torn Syria offer mute proof of the wisdom of fleeing conflict. The outpouring of a country's people into the Mediterranean and Europe has now been plugged back into Turkey, a country sinking rapidly into dictatorship.

Whole communities in the Yemen are being destroyed by Saudi missiles made in Britain. Yemeni children show the ginger hair and sticklike limbs of chronic malnutrition as this forgotten war continues. Russian warships cruise through the Mediterranean, ordered there by a leader who, as a young KGB officer posted to the East German town of Dresden, saw the Soviet Union collapse in 1989 and vowed to make it great again.

Under its current president, the Republic of South Africa, once a beacon of hope in the world, is increasingly enmeshed in greed and corruption. In the South China Sea, reefs that the waves idly washed over ten years ago have been raised into functioning military bases as the current Bejing government makes extraordinary new claims on international waters. The International Court in The Hague rules such claims illegal, but China's near neighbours are too nervous to press the point. European institutions, built out of the debris of two World Wars, show a new fragility after the people of the supposedly stable United Kingdom split 52:48 per cent in favour of leaving the European Union. The people of Europe feel a new fragility as terrorist attacks in their cities heighten any fear of foreigners.

Frustration grows for so many in society whose income has stalled, who know that the present establishment is not listening or caring about them. Nearly half the people of the UK, and now of America too, have awoken from a referendum or election night surprised by the country they previously felt at home in. Far right groups thrive in the unease and foster more fear. Together with Yeats, in his poem 'The Second Coming', we wonder what rough beasts may now be slouching towards Bethlehem to be born. We listen to the news and, despite our relative comfort and security, a miasma of fear pervades our lives. This fear affects us all. How best to meet it?

Do we cover the world with leather or do we put on a pair of shoes?

A man walking through wild terrain noticed how sharp the stones were on his feet and decided that the best way to deal with this problem would be to cover the land with leather so that nothing could prick his feet. He was hard at work on his gargantuan task when another man came along, smiled and said, 'Why don't you just make yourself a pair of leather shoes? Then you'll be able to walk freely anywhere.'

Starting, and continuing, gentle mindfulness and meditation practise is an extraordinarily effective pair of shoes to put on in troubled, jaggy times. It is *not* about hiding from global problems by sitting on a comfy meditation cushion. Rather, it is choosing to turn into and meet the real problem – our own alarm and fear. When we can bear to meet and listen to our own inner fear, something in us calms down, is comforted just by that very act of listening. Once we become calmer, less conflicted within ourselves, we are less easily frightened by other factors, be that a cancer diagnosis or the economic and political turmoil in the world. When we are calmer, we see more clearly and are less easily fooled by the fearmongers.

We are less easily led into war.

We discover that we have the capacity to tolerate, understand and live with the difficult – both within and without. We stop thinking that stress is bad for us and instead notice

I have the capacity to meet and deal with the challenge of stress. We may even notice, to our surprise, a calm strength coming up in us at times of stress. Most women who give birth are terrified beforehand, pretty bruised and battered during, but quietly amazed afterwards – by their own capacity. My overriding joy was in my baby, but I also had a quiet, smiley voice inside me for days after saying, *Wow, I didn't know this body could do that!*

Once we develop a healthy response to stress (one that's not foolhardy but is almost adventurous), we are no longer driven by an anxious need to take immediate control of any challenging situation. We reflect and respond instead of immediately reacting. As a result we do not frighten ourselves, or others, to the same extent. On assessing the situation in a calmer way we may choose to take very forceful action, but it will be we who decide what that action will be. By moving out of reactive fear within ourselves, we also move away from reactive hostility to others. We discover our capacity to live well not only with ourselves, but also with each other. Differences do not go away, but they are no longer automatically, reactively, interpreted as divisions to be feared and fought over.

Peace movements protesting against governments going to war always run the risk of becoming mirror images of the very aggression that they are protesting against. When, in 2003, we marched in Glasgow (as millions of others were doing in cities across globe) to protest against the forth-coming invasion of Iraq by Britain and the US, our quiet rural group was alongside some lively young Glaswegians. I understood and sympathised with their anger, but half an hour of marching beside them to the furious and endlessly repeated chant of 'What do we want? No war! When do we want it? Now!' was becoming wearisome for everyone within earshot. An elderly lady walking beside me waited until even the chanters themselves were becoming fatigued. Just after they had shouted for the hundredth time, 'What do we want? No war!', she sweetly turned to them and interjected, 'I suppose that would be peace, would it?' They grinned and dropped their battle cry. Timing is all.

If we fully practise peace and tolerance in our own lives, we can learn to live well together with unpredictability both internal and external; with uncertainty both local and global, with people of widely differing views, with health and sickness, with living and with dying. All lives include all of the above. We can pretend that our individual lives do not, but we will wear ourselves out in the process. Only once we allow our lives to be as full of joy and sorrow, safety and danger, certainty and unpredictability, birth and death as they really are, can we live freely – and magnificently.

Taking the risk of settling for more

I once listened to a Buddhist nun describe her own journey towards a deeper trust and love as rather akin to the way a young animal approaches the new and seemingly dangerous. She used as an example the behaviour of a friend's new kitten. The young kitten was fascinated by, but also nervous and shy of, this strange new visitor to the house in her long maroon robes. As the nun sat reading in her friend's house, she was amused to watch the young kitten's antics out of the corner of her eye. Sudden daring forays in her general direction were followed by the kitten rapidly darting back to a place of safety in the curtains, only to reappear and adventurously approach again. It was a game of curiosity versus terror in which curiosity would not let up. She noticed how each new foray brought the kitten closer and closer to her. She sat still. Finally, one foray brought the kitten so close that she simply reached out her hand, picked up the kitten and dropped it on to her lap – at which the kitten instantly relaxed, purred deeply and fell asleep. It was just where the kitten had wanted to be all along.

Adyashanti describes the journey of the seeker as being one of constantly knocking on the door, desperate to gain entry, then suddenly discovering that you've been knocking from the inside all along. Suddenly something yields, your perspective shifts and you see life from a different place. Then you begin to notice that you are not reacting to events in quite the same way. A situation that always used to vex you no longer does. Ancient grudges that you didn't even admit you had just don't seem to be active any more. Old cannonballs of destructive behaviour no longer get loaded and fired. This leaves a lot of space, for you and for your world.

Then you notice with wonder that you're less afraid, more trusting not only of life itself but of your way of living it. You feel much freer, you engage more, notice more and appreciate more. It's not that you know more – if anything, you know less. Yet a confidence that isn't entirely personal starts to come up in you. You directly see how so often our actions have stemmed from insecurity and fear, and have not lead to happiness. You are able to look more deeply and compassionately than you ever did before at how the whole painful cycle of isolation, loneliness, greed, fear and aggression feeds itself and perpetuates itself. 'The seeing is the doing'– and your old self is undone by it. [3]

Finding stability within the instability

One of my teachers is Lama Rinchen, a wonderful French woman who teaches on Holy Isle (off Arran, in Scotland). I saw her in 2006 when I was about to restart the drug tamoxifen, a recent scan having shown a slight regrowth of my tumour. I explained to her how happy I had been off the anti-oestrogen drug for the previous six months, how good I had been feeling in general, how steady my mood had been – and how my heart sank at the thought of returning to the edgy, angsty, premenstrual-like unstable mood I was always in after a few weeks back on tamoxifen. I told her how I dreaded being all over the place again; being calm and centred had felt so good.

She smiled and said, 'Ah yes, it is easy to become attached to stability.'

I was a bit thrown and asked, 'But isn't that the whole point – for the mind and mood to become more stable? What's wrong with enjoying that?'

'Nothing is wrong with enjoying that – it is enjoyable. But if we become *attached* to any state, even a calm state, we are less flexible, less able to be in the moment with whatever state appears. The attachment is the problem. The real challenge is to find the stability within the instability.'

As always on talking with Lama Rinchen, another chink of illumination slipped in past my blinkers. My view changed. I felt more relaxed about restarting the tamoxifen. I could even see it as an exercise: *was* there stability to be found within hormonal instability? I had certainly never found any as a young woman, but then I had never looked. I had never assumed that there might be a calm in the eye of the storm. And once Lama Rinchen said it, I saw that this quality was exactly what Akong Rinpoche and Lama Yeshe demonstrated: steadiness, calmness, continued ease and openness in the midst of tumultuous events that were utterly overwhelming the rest of us.

I saw that only a stability that remained in place under changing circumstance could truly be relied upon. And what intrigued me was the fact that those rare individuals who have this type of stability seem to be *more* engaged in the world, not less. Was that type of stability there in me? Not yet, for sure, but maybe a very tiny seed of it was there as a possibility, and my practice would be to water that seed and nurture it. That practice is ongoing as I stay on tamoxifen as I write. I do sense a deeper core stability slowly growing – often to be immediately lost, but that's okay too. It sure beats being constantly and irritably premenstrual at the stately age of sixty-four.

Just doing it

We all need to go at the pace that is right for us on this journey, remembering Thich Nhat Hanh's gentle advice to:

> *Maintain your health.*
> *Be joyful.*
> *Do not force yourself to do things you cannot do.* [4]

There are many excellent books on mindfulness and meditation. I give a list of titles that have helped me at the back of this book, and would recommend that anyone interested in beginning some regular meditation attend a nearby mindfulness or meditation course, or find an online course from an experienced teacher. It is really helpful to be part of a group who can support one another, and a good teacher is invaluable. Weekend courses at a recognised centre are particularly helpful. Research your options, and find the teacher you feel is right for you.

All that the much used term 'mindfulness' means is: 'Being aware of what is happening, when it is happening, no matter what it is' – the definition from Rob Nairn, precious teacher of mindfulness to so many. Mindfulness is a muscle we all already have. We do not have to go looking for it. We do not have to strive to invent it. We simply need to exercise it and strengthen it. The results can be remarkable if, in the gift of each present moment, we just do it.

In order to practice mindfulness and meditation I had to forget my perfect offering. I had to humbly discover how little I knew about anything, including my own mind. In order to write this book about my adventures in living with cancer, I have once again had to forget my perfect offering; as one friend said, that book wouldn't have been readable anyway.

This book has come about only through the generous and compassionate help of Chöje Lama Yeshe Losal Rinpoche, Abbot of Samye Ling Tibetan Buddhist monastery, and the help of many other wonderful teachers. It is dedicated to them all. May it be of benefit, in whatever way possible, to as many as possible.

Mary Gunn,
December 2016

References

Every effort has been made in the preparation of this book to provide correct and comprehensive references and to seek permission for the reproduction of any copyrighted quotations. Please contact the publisher if any error or omission is noted.

Foreword.

1 Jalāl ad-Dīn Muhammad Rūmī, translated by Coleman Barks, *Rumi: Selected Poems*, Penguin (2004). Reproduced here by kind permission of Coleman Barks

2 Appiah, Kwame Anthony, 'Mistaken Identities: Culture', BBC Reith Lectures (2016)

3 Gandhi, Mahatma, *The Collected Works of Mahatma Gandhi, Vol. 13, 1913*, Publications Division, Ministry of Information & Broadcasting, Government of India (1964)

Part 1: Three: Treatment.

1 Chödrön, Pema, *When Things Fall Apart*, Shambhala (1997)

2 Kübler-Ross, Elisabeth, *On Death and Dying*, Macmillan (1969)

Six: Recurrence, 2010

1 Nupen, Christopher, *Everything is a Present: The Wonder and Grace of Alice Sommer Herz*, Allegro Films (2010)

Well

Seven: A Skype Call to Mumbai

1 The American homeopath Dr Roger Morrison describes the Anacardium state as follows: 'There is a dichotomy inside the patient; he is pulled in two directions at once. The schism in the personality is expressed in our [homeopathic] literature ...: "Delusion of an angel on one shoulder, and the devil on the other" ... There can be pathological inferiority and low self-esteem.' Morrison, Roger, *Desktop Guide to Keynotes and Confirmatory Symptoms*. Hahnemann Clinic, 1993

2 Richard Feynman speaking in an interview on the BBC television programme *Horizon* (1981)

3 In 1928 Alexander Fleming was studying the staphylococcus bacteria in his London laboratory. That summer, before going on holiday with his family, Fleming had piled Petri dishes containing staphylo-coccal cultures to one side of his laboratory and left them without cleaning them out (these days he would be hauled over the Health and Safety coals by his line manager for such sloppy practice). It was a warm summer. On his return he noticed that a fungal spore, perhaps blown in through an open window, had contaminated one of the dishes. That dish contained a profuse growth of both staphylococci and an unknown fungus. But what Fleming noticed was that no staphylococcal colonies were growing adjacent to this fungus. There was an area clear of both fungus and staphylococcus. Fleming famously commented, 'That's funny', and went on to investigate the fungus further. He cultured it and found it produced a substance which killed many bacteria. The fungus was a penicil-lium mould, so Fleming named the substance he extracted from it 'penicillin'

Eight: Ways of Living with Dying

1 Vonnegut, Kurt, *Mother Night*, Dial Press Trade Paperbacks (1961)

2 Poem from the author's family collection

3 The scan showed a new, 4cm mass in the left lung: the cancer was indeed regrowing. A repeat CT scan six months later showed the mass to be the same size: no shrinkage, but no new growth either – for now, held stable on tamoxifen and a new homeopathic remedy

4 Poem from the author's family collection

Nine: Dying into Living

1 Mello, Anthony de, *Awareness*, Fount (1990)

2 Holub, Miroslav, translated by Ian Milner, *Poems Before and After:*

References

Collected English Translations, Bloodaxe Books (2006). www.
bloodaxebooks.com (reproduced here by kind permission of
Bloodaxe Books)

Part 2: One: How Do We Look at Our Life

1 Kant, Immanuel, translated by Paul Carus, *Prolegomena to Any Future
   Metaphysics,* CreateSpace (2017)

2 Löwel, S and Singer, W, 'Selection of intrinsic horizontal connections
   in the visual cortex by the correlated neuronal activity', *Science*,
   255 (1992)

3 Thinley Norbu, *A Cascading Waterfall of Nectar*, Shambhala (2006)

4 Katie, Byron, thework.com

5 Katie, Byron, thework.com

6 Gandhi, Mahatma, *The Collected Works of Mahatma Gandhi, Vol.
   13, 1913*, Publications Division, Ministry of Information &
   Broadcasting, Government of India (1964)

Two: You Cannot Step Twice Into the Same River.

1, 2 Graham, Daniel W, 'Heraclitus' in *Stanford Encyclopedia of Philosophy*,
   plato.stanford.edu (2017)

3 SN Goenka speaking in a video recording shown to course attendees
   at the Dhamma Dipa Vipassana Meditation Centre, Hereford

4 Brunschwig, J and Geoffrey ER Lloyd (Editors), *Greek Thought:
   A Guide to Classical Knowledge*, Harvard University Press (2000)

5 Popper, Karl, *World of Parmenides: Essays on the Presocratic Enlightenment*, Routledge (2012)

6 Keller, A, Litzelman, K Wisk LE *et al*, 'Does the perception that stress
   affects health matter? The association with health and mortality',
   Health Psychology, September 2012, 31 (5), 677–684

7 McGonigal, Kelly, 'How to make stress your friend', TED.com
   (2013)

8 Dzogchen Ponlop Rinpoche, *Mind Beyond Death*, Snow Lion
   (2012)

9, 10 Poems from the author's family collection

Three: What Increases Our Suffering and Lessens Our Happiness

1, 2 From the author's notes during a talk by Brother David Steindl-Rast at Sounds True, an event to celebrate the launch of The Eckhart Tolle Foundation, at Huntingdon Beach, California (September 29–October 2, 2016)

3 Flam, Jack (editor), *Matisse on Art*, University of California Press (1995)

4, 5 HH The Dalai Lama and Desmond Tutu, *The Book of Joy*, Hutchinson (2016)

6 Albert Einstein, quoted in the *New York Times* (May 25, 1946)

7 From a speech given by Martin Luther King Jr in St Louis, Missouri (March 22, 1964)

8 Richard Davidson speaking in an interview for www.onbeing.org with Kristen Tippet (June 23, 2011)

9 Mandela, Nelson, *Long Walk to Freedom: The Autobiography of Nelson Mandela*, Abacus (1995)

10 Ayele, Sophia, Fuentes-Nieva, Ricardo, Hardoon, Deborah, 'An Economy For the 1%: How privilege and power in the economy drive extreme inequality and how this can be stopped', Oxfam International (June 18, 2016)

11 Mandela, Nelson, *Long Walk to Freedom: The Autobiography of Nelson Mandela*, Abacus (1995)

Four: What Lessens Our Suffering and Increases Our Happiness

1, 2, 3 HH The Dalai Lama and Desmond Tutu, *The Book of Joy*, Hutchinson (2016)

Five: What Tools Do We Need To Effect These Changes?

1 Jalāl ad-Dīn Muhammad Rūmī, translated by Coleman Barks, *Rumi: Selected Poems*, Penguin (2004). Reproduced here by kind permission of Coleman Barks

2 'Tibet's Secret Temple', Wellcome Collection. London (November 15, 2016–February 28, 2016)

3 Nhat Hanh, Thich, *The Heart of the Buddha's Teaching*, Rider (1998)

4 Quote by Yongey Mingyur Rinpoche from the Introduction to: Ricard, Matthieu, *Why Meditate?*, Hay House (2010)

5 Kabat-Zinn, Jon, 'Mindfulness-Based Interventions in Context: Past,

References

Present, and Future', *Clinical Psychology Science in Practice*, 2003, Vol 10, Issue 2, 144–156

6 Ricard, Matthieu, *Why Meditate?*, Hay House (2010)

7 Tsoknyi Rinpoche, *Pundarika chant book*, Pundarika foundation
8 Dass, Ram, *Be Here Now*, Crown (1971)

9 Ram Dass speaking on a video featured on the 'Ram Dass Channel', YouTube

10 Quote by Yongey Mingyur Rinpoche from the Introduction to: Ricard, Matthieu, *Why Meditate?*, Hay House (2010)

Six: Many Paths, Same Destination

1 From the author's notes during a talk by Brother David Steindl-Rast at Sounds True, an event to celebrate the launch of The Eckhart Tolle Foundation, at Huntingdon Beach, California (September 29–October 2, 2016)

2 Nhat Hanh, Thich, *No Death, No Fear*, Rider (2002)

3 Nhat Hanh, Thich, *Understanding Our Mind*, Parallax (2006)

4 Feynman, Richard, *The Quotable Feynman*, Princeton University Press (2015)
5 Feynman, Richard, *Surely You're Joking, Mr Feynman!*, Bantam (1986)

6 Nhat Hanh, Thich, *Reconciliation, healing the inner child*, Parallax (2010)

7 Letter by Albert Einstein from 1950, as quoted in the *New York Times* (March 29, 1972) and the *New York Post* (November 28, 1972)

8 Einstein, Albert, *Science, Philosophy and Religion, A Symposium*, Conference on Science, Philosophy and Religion in Their Relation to the Democratic Way of Life, Inc., New York (1941)

9 Einstein, Albert, *The Human Side: New Glimpses From His Archives*, Princeton University Press (2013)

10 Feynman, Richard, *The Meaning of It All*, Perseus Books (1998)

11 From the Messenger Lectures at Cornell University, a talk entitled 'The Law of Gravitation, an Example of Physical Law' (1964)

12 Statement by Niels Bohr after the Solvay Conference of 1927, as quoted in Heisenberg, Werner, *Physics and Beyond*, Harper Collins (1971)

13 Anecdotal quote often attributed to Niels Bohr

Well

14 Schrödinger, Erwin, *Mind and Matter*, Cambridge University Press (1958)

15 Heisenberg, Werner, *Philosophic Problems of Nuclear Science*, Faber and Faber (1952)

16 Heisenberg, Werner, 'Scientific and Religious Truth' (1973)

17 Poem from the author's family collection

18 Qur'an 57:4

19 Qur'an 7:156

20 All three Jonathan Sacks quotes are from his official website, rabbisacks.org

21 Kononenko, Igor and Irena Roglic, *Teachers of Wisdom*, Dorrance Publishing (2010)

22 Sharma, Suresh K. and Usha, *Cultural and Religious Heriage of India: Sikhism*, Mittal publications (2004)

23 Melvyn, Roy, *The Four Taoist Classics*, Lulu Press, Inc (2012)

24, 25 Black Elk, 'The Sacred Pipe', quotes taken from Wikiquote

26 Nisargadatta, Sri Maharaj, *I Am That*, The Acorn Press (2005)

27 *The Complete Works of St Teresa of Jesus*, Sheed and Ward (1946)

28 Merton, Thomas, *New Seeds of Contemplation*, New Directions Publishing (2007)

29 From the author's notes whilst attending a retreat with Adya in the Netherlands (2016)

30 Jalāl ad-Dīn Muhammad Rūmī, translated by Coleman Barks, *Rumi: Selected Poems*, Penguin (2004)

Part 3: Love In a Time of Fear

1 HH The Dalai Lama, from the Samye Ling website (SamyeLing.org)

2 Nhat Hanh, Thich, *Understanding Our Mind*, Parallax (2006)

3 Krishnamurti, Jiddu, and Bohm, David, *The Limits of Thought: Discussions*, Routledge (1999)

4 Nhat Hanh, Thich, *The Heart of the Buddha's Teaching*, Rider (1998)

Useful Books

The following books have been very helpful to me, both in the writing of this book and in my life. It is by no means an exhaustive list but I hope that some of the titles may be of interest to the reader.

Adyashanti, *Falling into Grace*, Sounds True (2011)

Chödrön, Pema, *When Things Fall Apart*, Shambhala (1997)

HH The Dalai Lama and Desmond Tutu, *The Book of Joy*, Cornerstone Publishing (2016)

Kabat-Zinn, Jon, *Mindfulness for Beginners*, Sounds True (2012)

Kornfield, Jack, *A Path with a Heart*, Bantam Books (1993)

Lama Yeshe Rinpoche, *Living Dharma*, Dzalendra Publishing, Samye Ling (2001)

Mello, Anthony de, *Awareness*, Fount (1990)

Merton, Thomas, *New Seeds of Contemplation*, Shambhala (2003)

Nhat Hanh, Thich, *The Miracle of Mindfulness*, Rider (1975)

Nhat Hanh, Thich, *No Death, No Fear*, Rider (2002)

Nhat Hanh, Thich, *Living Buddha, Living Christ*, Rider (1995)

Nisargadatta, Sri Maharaj, *I Am That*, Acorn Press (2005)

Ricard, Matthieu, *Why Meditate?*, Hay House (2010)

Ringu Tulku, *Journey From Head to Heart*, Bodhicharya (2013)

Steindl-Rast, David, *Words of Common Sense*, Templeton Foundation Press (2002)

Suzuki Roshi, *Zen Mind, Beginner's Mind*, Weatherhill (2001)

Tsoknyi Rinpoche, *Open Heart, Open Mind*, Rider (2012)

Yongey Mingyur Rinpoche, *The Joy of Living*, Bantam Books (2009)

Acknowledgements

Thank you.

To the reader, for reaching this page, and to every single person whose story has woven its way into this book. To Sara Hunt of Saraband for her warm support throughout the publishing process, and to Craig Hillsley and Alex Newby whose careful editing has made this a much better book. To my friends at Samye Ling who constantly encouraged me to complete the book: Ani Yeshe Zangmo, Ani Sonam, Mimi Thomas and Mike Squire. To those who have kindly read parts of the book and given valuable feedback: Iain Bamforth, Val Beaver, Liz Findlay, Sandy and Susie Frame, Gavin Francis, Helen Hastings, Judy and Bob Johnstone, Iona and Laura Jones, Sarah MacIntyre, Caragh Morrish and her sister Shauna, Marian Newbery, Martha Reeves, Sandra Russell, Richard Smith, Jane and Derek Wooff. Especial thanks to Lama Rinchen who, as always, gave generously of her time and whose advice was invaluable. Heartfelt thanks to my husband John. He has not only had to live with a wife with cancer, but has patiently read all about it too. Hero status assured.

Well

Especial thanks to Coleman Barks for giving instant permission for his translations of Rumi's poems to be reproduced in the book; and to Suzanne Fairless-Aitken of Bloodaxe Books for permission to include Holub's poem 'The Door'. Such warm generosity of response buoyed me up just when I was beginning to sag under the detail of editing. Thank you too to Yeshe Lhadron, who kindly gave permission for her photo of Lama Yeshe on Holy Isle to be included in the book.

To my doctors and therapists, without whose expert care I would not have been here to write this book: my GPs over twenty years, Dr Bill Fiddes, Dr Dorothy Ainslie and Dr Alistair Wright; hospital consultants Dr Lillian Matheson, Mr John O'Neill, and Dr Carolyn Bedi; homeopathic consultants Dr Rajan Sankaran, Dr Julie Geraghty and Dr Bob Leckridge; and the therapists who gave invaluable support through all the times of adjustment, Nirved Wilson, Sue McLennan, Trevor Timms and Mike Wilson. To all the nurses who cared for me so well, and to the radiotherapy staff at the Western General Hospital, Edinburgh. Also thanks to the staff at the Maggie's Centre in Edinburgh and the Macmillan Centre at the Borders General Hospital. In ever more testing times, NHS patient care continues to be remarkable. To my GP partners who supported me getting back to work, and to all patients across all the years – thank you.

To my sister Donella – so often the wind in my sails. To all the dear friends who have been there for me on the end of a phone or ready with a cup of coffee. I do not mention you by name simply for fear of leaving one precious name out. But especial thanks to Judith Nicol and Diane Tasker, who listened through the hardest of times.

Acknowledgements

To my teachers over the years: Adyashanti, Akong Rinpoche, John Emery, Thich Nhat Hanh, Janet Heyes, Father MacLean, Sister Helen McLaughlin, Anthony de Mello, Mooji, Rob Nairn, Monsieur Perret-Gentil, Lama Rinchen, Ringu Tulku, David Steindl-Rast, Tsoknyi Rinpoche and Yongey Mingyur Rinpoche. My heartfelt thanks to Choje Lama Yeshe Losal Rinpoche, who inspired the writing of this book.

To my children and their partners who bring me such joy. To my husband who I love dearly. To my Dad for everything, and for his poems as well. To my Mum for being such fun, and for giving birth both to the title of this book and to its author.

Thank you. Thank you everyone.

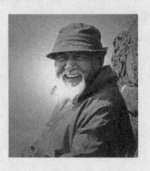

*To tame ourselves is the only way
we can change and improve the world.*

Choje Lama Yeshe Losal Rinpoche